Pharmanual

Emergir Pathogens: Implications for the Future

Editor
Robert C. Moellering, Jr, MD

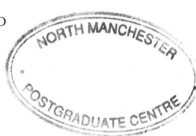
4 figures, 9 tables, 2001

℗ PharmaLibri

Montreal • Chicago

Pharmanual

Emerging Pathogens: Implications for the Future

Editor: Robert C. Moellering, Jr, MD
ISBN 0-919839-56-8

Pharmanual is a registered trademark

Library of Congress Cataloging-in-Publication Data

Emerging pathogens : implications for the future / editor, Robert C. Moellering, Jr.
　　p. ; cm. — (Pharmanual)
　　Includes bibliographical references.
　　ISBN 0-919839-56-8 (pbk.)
　　1. Drug resistance in microorganisms. 2. Vancomycin resistance. I. Moellering, Robert C. II Pharmanual (Chicago, Ill.)
　　[DNLM: 1. Drug Resistance, Microbial. 2. Clostridium difficile—drug effects. 3. Enterococcus—drug effects. 4. Enterocolitis, Pseudomembranous. 5. Vancomycin Resistance. 6. Beta-Lactam Resistance. WB 330 E53 2000]
　　QR177.E44 2000
　　616'.01—dc21

00-055764

Drug Dosage
　　The authors and the publisher have exerted every effort to ensure that drug selection and dosage set forth in this text are in accord with current recommendations and practice at the time of publication. However, in view of ongoing research, changes in government regulations, and the constant flow of information relating to drug therapy and drug reactions, the reader is urged to check the product labeling for each drug for any change in indications and dosage and for added warnings and precautions. This is particularly important when the recommended agent is a new and/or infrequently employed drug.

© Copyright 2001 by
PharmaLibri Publishers, Inc., 2222 René-Lévesque W, Montreal, Quebec, Canada, H3H 1R6.
Printed in the UK.
ISBN 0-919839-56-8

Contents

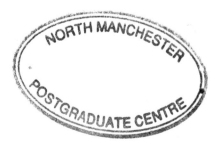

I.   Emergence of Pathogenic Resistance

Robert C. Moellering, Jr

A national surveillance study in the United States reported that 0.3% of enterococcal isolates exhibited resistance to vancomycin in 1989 [1]. By 1993, that percentage had increased to 7.9%. In intensive care units, the situation was more dramatic, with the incidence increasing from 0.4% to 13.6%. Of further concern, reports have documented that strains of vancomycin-resistant enterococci (VRE) have spread between hospitals, and the expression of this resistance has been seen in multiple strains of bacteria [2-4]. More than 10% of strains of *Klebsiella pneumoniae* in the United States have been estimated to produce extended-spectrum beta-lactamases (ESBLs), and a global surveillance program has estimated that 20% of *K pneumoniae* produce ESBLs worldwide [5, Ron Jones, personal communication, SENTRY Antimicrobial Surveillance Program, 1997 and 1998, University of Iowa].

Compounding this problem of growing resistance among prominent pathogens are the increasingly limited therapeutic options available for treating infection caused by VRE or ESBL-producing bacilli. As noted by Curtis J. Donskey, MD, and Louis B. Rice, MD, in this volume, enterococci are intrinsically resistant to cephalosporins, penicillinase-resistant penicillins, aztreonam, clindamycin, trimethoprim-sulfamethoxazole, and clinically achievable levels of aminoglycosides, eliminating these agents as treatment options for monotherapy [4]. Further, VRE not only are resistant to vancomycin, but they have exhibited resistance to penicillin, erythromycin, tetracycline, and high levels of aminoglycosides, and they can be resistant to all currently available antibiotics used for treatment of vancomycin-susceptible enterococci. Jan E. Patterson, MD, points out that ESBLs confer various degrees of resistance to broad-spectrum cephalosporins, aztreonam, and extended-spectrum penicillins. They also may be resistant to beta-lactamase inhibitor combinations, fluoroquinolones, aminoglycosides, and carbapenems. Further, resistance determinants to other antibacterials often are cotransferred on a resistance plasmid, which results in multiple drug resistance [6,7].

Detection of resistant strains also presents a problem with VRE and ESBLs. Drs. Donskey and Rice note that automated susceptibility testing methods may not correctly identify those strains of VRE that have relatively low levels of vancomycin resistance. Dr. Patterson points out that ESBL-producing gram-negative bacilli may appear susceptible at a standard inoculum of 10^5, but minimum inhibitory concentrations can be significantly elevated at higher inocula of 10^7 or 10^8, which are seen with certain third- and "fourth"-generation cephalosporins.

All of these factors combine to present a grave problem in treating infections that commonly occur among seriously ill, debilitated patients. Numerous measures have been undertaken in an attempt to control outbreaks and the spread of resistant pathogens. Strict isolation precautions, surveillance of antibiotic usage patterns, selective restriction of antibiotics known to be associated with these two types of resistance, and limiting the duration of empiric therapy all have been employed with varying degrees of success.

Yet another concern related to antibiotic resistance is the emergence of *Clostridium difficile*-associated pseudomembranous colitis, as chronicled by Donald E. Fry, MD, in this volume. This pathogen has become the most common cause of infectious, hospital-acquired diarrhea [8], and prior administration of antibiotics, which is believed to disrupt normal colonization resistance in the gut, has been documented in more than 90% of cases of emerging *C difficile* infection [9]. The antibiotics associated most commonly with the development of this infection are ampicillin, amoxicillin, clindamycin, and the cephalosporins. Antifungal, antiviral, and antineoplastic chemotherapy also have been associated with *C difficile* infection. As with VRE and ESBL-producing bacilli, patients at greatest risk appear to be those who are severely ill and debilitated. Adding to the resistance problem is that one of the primary agents recommended for treatment of *C difficile* infection is vancomycin, whose unrestricted use could contribute further to the development and spread of VRE.

Infection control measures for *C difficile* pseudomembranous colitis focus on disinfection and cleaning policies, selective restriction of antibiotics that are strongly associated with enterocolitis, and limiting the duration of antibiotic therapy.

Emerging antibiotic resistance among nosocomial pathogens presents an ongoing challenge to infectious disease specialists. The limited therapeutic options available to clinicians treating a seriously ill, particularly susceptible patient population underline the gravity of the situation. Although we must continue intensive efforts to investigate and develop treatment alternatives, the most effective strategies at present appear to be strict measures designed to prevent and control the spread of these deadly microorganisms and programs to foster appropriate use of antimicrobial agents.

References

1. Centers for Disease Control and Prevention. Nosocomial enterococci resistant to vancomycin-United States, 1989-1993. *MMWR Morbid Mort Week Rep.* 1993;42:597-599.
2. Chow JW, Kuritza A, Shlaes DM, Green M, Sahm DF, Zervos MJ. Clonal spread of vancomycin resistant *Enterococcus faecium* between patients in three hospitals in two states. *J Clin Microbiol.* 1993;31:1609-1611.
3. Donskey CJ, Schreiber JR, Jacobs MR, et al. A polyclonal outbreak of predominantly VanB vancomycin-resistant enterococci in Northeast Ohio. *Clin Infect Dis.* 1999;29:573-579.
4. Morris JG, Shay DK, Hebden JN, et al. Enterococci resistant to multiple antimicrobial agents, including vancomycin: establishment of endemicity in a university medical center. *Ann Intern Med.* 1995;123:250-259.
5. Fridkin SK, Gaynes RP. Antimicrobial resistance in intensive care units. *Clin Chest Med.* 1999;20:303-316.
6. Sader HS, Pfaller MA, Jones RN. Prevalence of important pathogens and the antimicrobial activity of parenteral drugs at numerous medical centers in the United States. II. Study of the intra- and interlaboratory dissemination of extended-spectrum beta-lactamase-producing *Enterobacteriaceae*. *Diagn Microbiol Infect Dis.* 1994;20:203-208.
7. Gazouli M, Kaufmann ME, Tzelepi E, Dimopoulou H, Paniara O, Tzouvelekis LS. Study of an outbreak of cefoxitin-resistant *Klebsiella pneumoniae* in a general hospital. *J Clin Microbiol.* 1997;35:508-510.
8. Ringel AF, Jameson GL, Foster ES. Diarrhea in the intensive care patient. *Crit Care Clin.* 1995;11:465-477.
9. Vollaard EJ, Clasener HAL, van Saene HKF, et al. Effect of colonization resistance: an important criterion in selecting antibiotics. *DICP: Anu Pharmacother.* 1990;24:60-66.

Robert C. Moellering, Jr, MD, Herman Blumgart Professor of Medicine, Harvard Medical School, Physician-in-Chief, Beth Israel Deaconess Medical Center, Boston, Massachusetts, USA.

II. Vancomycin Resistance in Enterococci

Curtis J. Donskey and Louis B. Rice

Introduction

The first clinical strains of vancomycin-resistant enterococci (VRE) were reported in 1988. Since that time, these organisms have rapidly emerged as important nosocomial pathogens, particularly in the United States. Infection control measures have not been effective in preventing the spread of VRE, although such initiatives may limit the size of outbreaks. In addition, experience suggests that the development of new antimicrobial agents in response to the threat of VRE will provide only a temporary solution. The purpose of this chapter is to review enterococcal infections, mechanisms and epidemiology of vancomycin resistance, and potential control measures, including selective use of antibiotics.

Enterococcal Infections

Enterococci are components of the normal intestinal flora of humans and animals. They are hardy, facultative anaerobes that can survive and grow in a variety of environments; they have been isolated from soil, water, and food samples. In hospital settings, enterococci have been cultured from environmental surfaces and from the hands of healthcare workers [1]. *Enterococcus faecalis* is the most prevalent species cultured from humans, accounting for 80% to 90% of clinical isolates [2], and in recent years, isolation of *E faecium* strains that are resistant to multiple antibiotics has become increasingly common in the hospital setting [3]. Fifteen other species of enterococci are currently recognized, but only *E faecalis and E faecium* are commonly associated with clinical infection [4].

Infections typically caused by enterococci include endocarditis, bacteremia, urinary tract infection, wound infection, and intra-abdominal and pelvic infections. Many infecting strains originate from the patient's intestinal flora, which can spread and cause urinary tract, intra-abdominal, and surgical wound infections. Bacteremia may result, with seeding of more distant sites. For example, genitourinary tract infection or instrumentation often precedes the onset of enterococcal endocarditis [5]. Person-to-person spread of enterococcal strains has been suggested by molecular epidemiologic analysis, but it is generally accepted that in most of these cases, the acquired strains become part of the colonizing flora before they cause serious clinical infection.

Enterococci have emerged as an important cause of nosocomial infections during the past two decades. In recent National Nosocomial Infections Surveillance (NNIS) surveys in the United States, enterococci have ranked from the second to the fourth most common cause of nosocomial infections, with particular prominence as causes of urinary tract, bloodstream, and wound infections [6]. This increasing prominence of enterococci as nosocomial pathogens may be due in part to a general increase in the severity of illness among hospitalized patients and to frequent use of indwelling vascular and urinary catheters. Nosocomial enterococcal infections typically occur in very ill, debilitated patients who have been exposed to broad-spectrum antibiotics. The ability of enterococci to thrive in the presence of intense antibiotic pressure in the hospital environment also has contributed to their emergence as nosocomial pathogens.

Antibiotic Resistance in Enterococci

Enterococci are intrinsically resistant to cephalosporins, penicillinase-resistant penicillins, aztreonam, clindamycin, trimethoprim-sulfamethoxazole, and clinically achievable levels of aminoglycosides (Table II-1) [2]. Compared with most streptococcal species, enterococci are also relatively resistant to penicillin, with minimum inhibitory concentrations (MICs) generally ranging from 2 to 8 mg/mL for *E faecalis* and 8 to 32 mg/mL for *E faecium*. The intrinsic resistance of *E faecium* to penicillin is due to the expression of the cell wall synthesis enzyme PBP5 (a low-affinity penicillin-binding protein) [7]. In addition, enterococci exhibit tolerance to the action of all cell wall-active antibiotics, including penicillins and vancomycin. Therefore, enterococci will be inhibited, but not killed, when exposed to these agents. Synergistic bactericidal activity against enterococci can be achieved only by combining a cell wall-active agent with an aminoglycoside. For serious infections such as endocarditis, achieving bactericidal activity by combining penicillin with streptomycin was associated with a doubling of the cure rate from 40% to 80% [8-10].

Table II-1. Mechanisms of Antimicrobial Resistance in Enterococci

Antibiotic	Mechanism of Resistance
Intrinsic resistance	
β-lactams	Decreased affinity of lower-weight penicillin-binding proteins (especially PBP5)
Aminoglycosides	Low-level resistance due to decreased permeability
Trimethoprim-sulfamethoxazole	In vivo resistance due to ability to use exogenous folates
Lincosamides	Chromosomal low-level resistance
Vancomycin	Low-level resistance (*E gallinarum* and *E casseliflavus*) due to production of altered peptidoglycan precursors
Acquired resistance	
All cell wall-active agents	Tolerance
β-lactams	β-lactamase production
	Altered PBPs
Aminoglycosides	Modifying enzymes
	Ribosomal mutation (streptomycin only)
Fluoroquinolones	DNA gyrase mutation
Tetracycline	Increase efflux of drug
Rifampin	DBA-dependent RNA polymerase mutation
Chloramphenicol	Chloramphenicol acetyltransferase
Macrolides/ Lincosamides/ Streptogramins	Reduced ribosomal binding due to methylation of rRNA
Vancomycin	High-level resistance (VanA and VanB) due to production of altered peptidoglycan precursors with decreased affinity for vancomycin

Their prominent representation in normal human bowel flora ensures that enterococci are exposed to all antibiotics excreted through the gastrointestinal tract. This persistent selective pressure has been associated with the progressive acquisition by enterococci of determinants conferring resistance to many intrinsically active antibiotic classes, including penicillin (by β-lactamase production), erythromycin, tetracycline, high levels of aminoglycosides, and vancomycin (Table II-1) [2]. Particularly important among these resistance phenotypes is

Table II-2. Types of Vancomycin Resistance in Enterococci

Phenotype/Genotype	Expression	Transfer	MIC (mg/mL) Vancomycin	Teicoplanin	Species
VanA/vanA	inducible	+	64->1,024	16-512	E. faecium E. faecalis E. avium (rare) E. durans (rare)
VanB/vanB	inducible	+	4-1,000	0.5-1.0	E. faecium E. faecalis
VanC/vanC1 and vanC2	constitutive	-	2-32	0.5-1.0	E. gallinarum E. casseliflavus
VanD/vanD	constitutive	-	64	4	E. faecium
VanE/vanE	constitutive	-	16	0.5	E. faecalis

MIC = minimum inhibitory concentration

resistance to high levels of aminoglycoside. Conferred by the elaboration of aminoglycoside-modifying enzymes, high-level resistance results in a loss of bactericidal synergism that normally is associated with penicillin-aminoglycoside combinations. Although large studies are not available, it appears that the in vitro loss of synergism translates into an important clinical effect, as suggested by more common failures of medical therapy in these settings. High-level gentamicin-resistant enterococcal strains are now widespread in hospitals in the United States, and strains resistant to high levels of both gentamicin and streptomycin are being seen with increased frequency [11]. Penicillin resistance due to production of β-lactamase has been described, but it has not become widespread and has not had a significant impact on the ability to treat clinical infections where it has appeared. In contrast, high-level penicillin resistance due to production of altered PBPs is becoming increasingly common and is associated with important clinical effects [12].

The acquisition of vancomycin resistance by enterococci has had serious implications for the treatment and infection control of these organisms. VRE, particularly *E faecium* strains, are often resistant to all antibiotics effective for treatment of vancomycin-susceptible enterococci. The result is that clinicians are left with either suboptimal bacteriostatic agents such as chloramphenicol or with no therapeutic options to treat VRE infections. The potential for transfer of vancomycin-resistance genes from enterococci to *Staphylococcus aureus,* which has been achieved in vitro but has yet to be reported in the clinical setting, increases the importance of finding ways to limit the spread of VRE.

Mechanisms of Glycopeptide Resistance

Vancomycin is a member of the glycopeptide class of antibiotics. The only other glycopeptide available for clinical use is teicoplanin, an antibiotic licensed in Europe but not available in the United States. Glycopeptide antibiotics inhibit bacterial cell wall synthesis by binding to D-alanyl-D-alanine (D-ala-D-ala) at the terminus of a pentapeptide precursor involved in peptidoglycan synthesis. Under normal circumstances, this pentapeptide precursor is bound by the transpeptidases responsible for cross-linking the peptide chains of the peptidoglycan. By binding to the D-ala-D-ala terminus of the pentapeptide precursor, vancomycin prevents the cross-linking reaction [13]. In addition, it is believed that the bulky nature of vancomycin results in inhibition of transglycosylation. Cell wall synthesis, therefore, is inhibited, and the bacteria eventually lyse. Although the multiple genetic and enzymatic events involved in conferring vancomycin resistance are complicated, the ultimate basis for resistance is surprisingly simple; a peptidoglycan precursor with an altered pentadepsipeptide terminus, primarily

D-ala-D-lactate, is produced [13]. Vancomycin binds D-ala-D-lactate with much lower affinity than D-ala-D-ala, while PBPs appear to bind it without difficulty, thereby allowing cell wall synthesis to proceed (apparently) normally. Almost all bacteria synthesize peptidoglycan terminating in D-ala-D-ala, but clinically available glycopeptides inhibit only gram-positive bacteria because these molecules are larger than the exclusion limits of the porin proteins found in gram-negative outer membranes [14].

Five phenotypes of vancomycin resistance, termed VanA, VanB, VanC, VanD, and VanE, have been described (Table II-2) [5]. The VanA and VanB phenotypes are clinically significant and are mediated by one of two acquired, transferable operons consisting of seven genes, termed the VANA and VANB operons (Fig. II-1). These gene clusters were reported initially in enterococcal strains in 1988. The VanA resistance phenotype is the most common reported in the United States and Europe. VanA enterococcal isolates exhibit high-level resistance to both vancomycin and teicoplanin; VanB isolates have variable resistance to vancomycin and remain susceptible to teicoplanin. The VanC phenotype is mediated by chromosomal *vanC1 and vanC2* genes that are constitutively present in *E gallinarum (vanC1)* and *E casseliflavus (vanC2)* [5]. These genes confer relatively low levels of resistance to vancomycin and are not transferable. The VanD phenotype has been described only in a single strain of *E faecium* that had constitutive resistance to vancomycin (MIC, 64 mg/mL) and low levels of teicoplanin

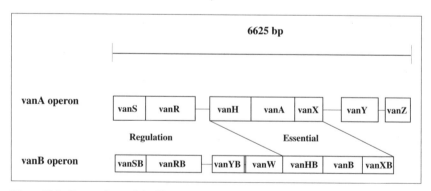

Figure II-1. Comparison of the VanA and VanB vancomycin resistance operons. The vanH, vanA, and vanX genes encode proteins that are essential for expression of vancomycin resistance in VanA-type VRE. These genes correlate with vanHB, vanB, and vanXB genes in VanB-type VRE. bp = base pairs.

(MIC, 4 mg/mL) [15]. The VanE phenotype has been described in a single strain of *E faecalis* that expressed constitutive resistance to vancomycin (MIC, 16 mg/mL), but was susceptible to teicoplanin [16]. The VanE phenotype is biochemically and phenotypically similar to the VanC phenotype.

The genetic basis for vancomycin resistance is best described for VanA-type VRE [13]. The *vanS* and *vanR* genes encode proteins (VanS and VanR) that are involved in induction of resistance. VanS functions as a sensor to detect the presence of vancomycin. VanR, the response regulator, activates transcription of three genes *(vanH, vanA, and vanX)* that encode proteins essential for the expression of vancomycin resistance. VanH is a dehydrogenase that converts pyruvate to D-lactic acid. VanA is a ligase that ligates D-lactate with D-alanine to form D-ala-D-lac. D-ala-D-lac is added to a tripeptide precursor by the cellular-adding enzyme to form a pentadepsipeptide precursor for cell wall peptidoglycan synthesis. VanX is a dipeptidase that cleaves the dipeptide D-ala-D-ala, thereby reducing the amount of normal dipeptide precursor available for incorporation into the pentapeptide precursors. VanY, not essential for expression of resistance, is a carboxypeptidase that cleaves the terminal D-ala from the normal pentapeptide. Because cleavage of the terminal D-alanine is the source of energy required for the transpeptidation reaction, these precursors will be ineffective. The function of VanZ is not known, and this protein is not required for expression of vancomycin resistance.

VanB-type vancomycin resistance is genetically and functionally similar to VanA-type resistance. The genes involved in VanB-type resistance share considerable sequence identity with the *vanA* genes [14]. Both resistance types result in the production of the same altered pentadepsipeptide precursor ending in D-ala-D-lac.

Spread of Vancomycin Resistance Determinants

Although early reports of VRE outbreaks commonly attributed spread to the transmission of specific resistant clones [17], in more recent and mature outbreaks, several clones have been identified when endemic VRE have been genotyped [18]. The existence of multiple clones implies mechanisms for the transmission of vancomycin resistance determinants between different organisms. Molecular analysis of regions flanking the vancomycin resistance operons has revealed several transposons that confer mobility to these determinants. The VanA operon is most commonly located within a Tn*3*-family transposon designated Tn*1546* [19]. This 10.6-kb element is found almost universally in association with VanA, although the restriction map will differ depending upon whether and where IS elements have inserted into the transposon. Tn*1546* has been shown to be mobile in enterococci, and it is thought that its ability to move between enterococcal strains is due to its integration into conjugative plasmids.

To date, two transposons have been associated with the VanB operon. Tn*1547* has been described in only a single strain of *E faecalis* [20]. It is approximately 60 kb in size and owes its mobility to the presence of IS*256*-like insertion elements on its ends. A more commonly found transposon in VanB *E faecium* strains is Tn*5382* [12]. This transposon is approximately 28 kb and has features similar to those of the well-characterized conjugative transposons. Tn*5382* can excise from the *E faecium* chromosome, but it has not been shown to be conjugative by itself. It does move with some frequency between *E faecium* strains as a component of a larger transferable element that also encodes PBP5-mediated ampicillin resistance. It appears likely that chromosome-to-chromosome transfer explains most observed VanB dissemination, although plasmid-mediated VanB has been described in rare cases [21].

Origin of Vancomycin Resistance Determinants

Examination of chromosomal DNA sequences from streptomycetes that are the natural producers of glycopeptide antibiotics *(Amycolatopsis orientalis, Actinomyces teicomyceticus)* suggests that these operons are derived from natural producers of the antibiotics [22]. The long delay between the clinical introduction of vancomycin and the appearance of resistance determinants in enterococci remains unexplained, but it may be due to the practice, begun in the United States in the early 1980s, of treating *Clostridium difficile*-induced diarrhea with orally administered vancomycin. This probably led to colonization by these glycopeptide producers and eventual transfer of the resistance determinants to the enterococci.

Epidemiology of Vancomycin Resistance

The first strains of VRE were reported in England in 1988 [23]. In the United States, VRE were first reported in New York City in 1989 [24]. Subsequently, VRE have rapidly spread throughout the United States. From 1989 to 1993, the NNIS reported that the percentage of enterococcal isolates exhibiting vancomycin resistance increased from 0.3% to 7.9% [3]. During the same time period, the percentage of enterococcal isolates exhibiting vancomycin resistance from intensive care units increased from 0.4% to 13.6%. VRE were initially isolated primarily in large university hospitals, but recent reports have documented significant VRE outbreaks in community hospitals and chronic care facilities [25].

VRE in the United States Versus Europe

In the United States, VRE have been isolated almost exclusively from hospitalized (or recently hospitalized) individuals. A study in Texas found no VRE isolates in human volunteers who had no exposure to hospitals [5]. Studies of stool samples from farm animals and chicken carcasses or feces in the United States have not found isolates of VRE. Of note, however, is a recent report of a VanB VRE strain isolated from a bag of chicken feed in the United States [26].

In early reports in the United States, hospital-associated VRE outbreaks often were due to dissemination of single strains of VRE, and infection control measures were successful in controlling the outbreaks [17]. Spread of VRE strains between hospitals in individual cities and between three hospitals in two states also has been reported [27]. More recent outbreaks have been characterized by expression of vancomycin resistance by multiple strains, suggesting spread of vancomycin-resistance determinants between strains of enterococci [18,28]. In several of these polyclonal outbreaks, infection control measures were unable to eliminate VRE from the hospital, although these measures may limit increases in the prevalence of colonization [18,28].

In contrast to the United States, there appears to be a large community reservoir of VRE in Europe. VanA-type VRE have been isolated from various farm animals, chicken carcasses, and other meat products as well as waste water samples from sewage treatment plants [5]. In a German community, 12% (12/100) of healthy persons screened in 1994 were found to be carriers of VRE [29]. In Belgium, van der Auwera et al [30] found that 28% of healthy community volunteers who had no known glycopeptide exposure were colonized with VRE.

The use of avoparcin, a glycopeptide antibiotic, as a growth promoter for farm animals has been proposed as an explanation for the epidemiology of VRE in Europe. This antibiotic has been used in some European countries since the 1970s and would have provided a selective pressure for the emergence and spread of vancomycin resistance genes. This hypothesis is supported by a Danish study that documented VanA-type VRE in chicken stool samples from farms using avoparcin, but not in samples from farms that did not use it [31]. Klare et al [29] found that after avoparcin use in animal husbandry was discontinued in Germany, the prevalence of VRE fecal colonization in healthy individuals in the Saxony-Anhalt region decreased from 12% to 3%, concurrent with a similar decrease in the prevalence of VRE in German poultry products. van den Bogaard et al [32] have demonstrated the presence of an identical VanA-VRE strain in a turkey farmer and his flock.

Although commonly isolated from healthy individuals in Europe, VRE has been less important as a nosocomial pathogen in Europe than in the United States

[5]. The reason for this phenomenon is not known. It has been proposed that aggressive control of other gram-positive pathogens, such as methicillin-resistant *Staphylococcus aureus*, may have had the unintended but beneficial consequence of limiting the spread of nosocomial VRE in some European countries [14]. Alternatively, it is conceivable that the Europeans have benefited from their use of avoparcin. Comparison of antimicrobial susceptibility data in VRE isolated from Europe and the United States reveals that, while virtually all of the United States isolates express resistance to high levels of ampicillin, only 33% of European isolates do so. These data suggest that the genetic exchange that led to the creation of VRE in Europe (in the lumen of healthy animal gastrointestinal tracts) occurred in an entirely different enterococcal population than in the United States, where VRE resulted from genetic exchange events in the gastrointestinal tracts of severely ill patients. It was well recognized even before the widespread emergence of VRE in the United States that the endemic population of *E faecium* in hospitals in this country was becoming more resistant to ampicillin. Selecting for transfer of vancomycin resistance determinants to strains already highly adapted for survival in the hospital environment may have inadvertently caused a more severe and extensive VRE outbreak.

VRE in Cleveland, Ohio

A molecular epidemiologic analysis of a large VRE outbreak in Cleveland, Ohio [28] illustrates several features common to VRE outbreaks in the United States as well as features unique to this geographic area. VRE initially were reported in the city in 1992, and several hospitals in the area were reporting significant rates of VRE colonization and infection by 1994. We studied the molecular epidemiology of VRE strains isolated in Cleveland-area hospitals during 1996. More than 300 VRE isolates from 13 hospitals were analyzed. Pulsed-field gel electrophoresis (PFGE) revealed 30 different strains, with one strain (PFGE Type A) present in all hospitals and seven strains present in three or more hospitals (Table II-3). In addition, analysis of VRE strains isolated from patients in a number of area nursing homes revealed the presence of several outbreak strains, including the predominant strain (PFGE Type A), which was seen in all of the nursing homes. Susceptibility testing and polymerase chain reaction assay of vancomycin resistance genes indicated that 79% of strains expressed the VanB phenotype and 21% expressed the VanA phenotype.

This outbreak illustrates the rapid emergence of VRE as a significant nosocomial pathogen in many hospitals in one geographic region. The presence of one predominant VRE strain among all of the hospitals and nursing homes analyzed and of seven strains in three or more hospitals suggests the transfer of

Table II-3. Pulsed-field Gel Electrophoresis of Vancomycin-resistant Enterococci from 12 Hospitals in Northeast Ohio

Hospital	A	B	C	D	E	F	H	I	J	K	L	M	N	Q	R	U	Total
1	7	.	.	.	1	.	.	.	.	1	.	.	1	.	.	2	12
2	48	3	9	2	31	.	3	.	.	.	7	2	1	.	.	5	111
3	25	.	10	.	.	.	.	.	.	.	.	1	.	.	1	.	36
4	64	.	13	2	1	1	.	2	6	4	1	2	.	1	1	.	97
5	2	.	.	.	.	.	.	.	.	.	.	2	.	.	.	1	20
6	25	1	2	.	2	.	.	.	.	.	6	3	.	1	.	2	41
7	2	.	.	.	.	.	.	.	.	.	.	.	.	.	.	.	2
8	11	.	.	.	.	.	.	.	.	.	1	.	.	.	.	.	12
9	8	.	1	.	5	1	.	.	2	.	1	.	.	.	.	.	18
10	3	.	.	.	.	.	.	.	.	.	.	.	.	.	.	.	3
11	1	1	.	.	.	.	.	.	.	.	.	.	.	.	.	.	2
12	1	.	.	.	.	.	.	.	.	.	1	.	.	.	.	.	2
13	1	.	1	.	5	.	.	.	.	.	.	.	.	.	.	.	7
Total	198	8	36	4	44	2	3	2	9	5	21	10	2	2	2	15	363

A-R represents different pulsed-field electrophoresis genotypes with more than one member.
U represents unique pulsed-field gel electrophoresis genotypes.
Reprinted with permission from Donskey CJ et al. [28].

individual strains between patients and ultimately between healthcare facilities. Trick et al [25] recently reported a large VRE outbreak in the Sioux City, Iowa, area in which similar evidence was found for spread of related strains between three acute care hospitals and several local chronic care facilities. A case-control study revealed that chronic care facility patients with VRE colonization were significantly more likely than VRE-negative controls to have been recent inpatients at an acute care facility [25].

The presence of many different VRE strains with VanB-type vancomycin resistance in a limited area was an unusual feature of the Cleveland-area outbreak. Most VanB outbreaks have been due to spread of one VRE strain. This observation may be attributable to the fact that the VanB resistance operon is most often chromosomal and transferable only at low frequency. Further analysis of different VanB strains from the Cleveland area resulted in identification of a large, transferable, mobile element that encodes both the vanB operon and a low-affinity *pbp5* gene (encoding high-level ampicillin resistance) [12]. The transfer of this large element between enterococci appears to be a primary reason for the genotypic variability of the VRE in the region, and it may be promoted by antibiotic pressure.

Presence of Vancomycin Resistance Genes in Nonenterococcal Species

It is somewhat surprising that the vancomycin resistance determinants remain largely restricted to enterococcal species. There is ample evidence for the presence of identical resistance determinants for several antibiotics, including chloramphenicol, erythromycin, gentamicin, mercuric chloride, and tetracycline, in enterococci, streptococci, and staphylococci. Although a major concern since their emergence has been the possibility that vancomcyin resistance determinants would migrate into staphylococci, no such strain ever has been observed in the clinical setting, although such an exchange has been accomplished in the laboratory. To date, of clinically important human pathogens, only a single VanB-encoding *Streptococcus bovis* strain has been described [33].

Importance of Intestinal Colonization in Spread of VRE

The intestinal tract is the most important source for spread of VRE (Fig. II-2). Most patients harboring VRE have asymptomatic intestinal colonization that may persist for months [34]. These individuals are at risk for developing infection with VRE and are a potential source for spread of these strains to the hands of healthcare workers, to the environment, and to other patients. Patients who have higher concentrations of VRE in their feces present a potentially greater risk for spread of VRE [5].

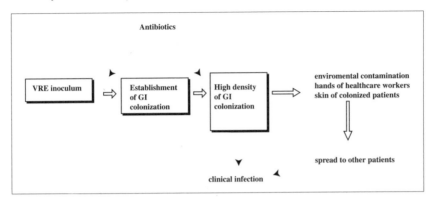

Figure II-2. The role of gastrointestinal colonization in the spread of VRE. Antibiotics may positively or negatively influence the establishment of VRE colonization and/or the density of colonization. Other factors also may affect intestinal colonization and the development of clinical infection (see text). Reprinted with permission from Donskey and Rice [44].

Because exposure to VRE strains is important for the development of colonization, factors that increase the likelihood of exposure (such as proximity to patients colonized with VRE) will increase the risk of colonization. Exposure to antibiotics is a major factor that promotes the establishment of VRE intestinal colonization and growth of VRE to high levels in the intestinal tract. Other factors that determine whether colonization is established after exposure to VRE and the level of established colonization are less clear.

Risk Factors for VRE Colonization and Infection
Risk factors for VRE colonization and infection have been derived from several case-control and cohort studies. The conclusions that can be drawn from many of these individual studies are limited because small numbers of cases were analyzed. Comparisons between studies are also limited because different outcomes were evaluated in many studies. For example, some studies have evaluated risk factors for colonization, while others have assessed risk factors for infection or bacteremia. Despite these limitations, many factors have been associated with VRE colonization and infection in multiple studies. Both nonantimicrobial and antimicrobial risk factors have been identified.

Nonantimicrobial risk factors for VRE colonization or infection include length of hospital stay, proximity to other patients colonized or infected with VRE, nonisolated intensive care unit days of care, and increased severity of illness [4]. These factors obviously may increase the likelihood of exposure to VRE strains. Edmond et al [35] found that the development of VRE bacteremia in oncology patients was associated with prior intestinal colonization. Shay et al [36] found that VRE bacteremia was associated with increased severity of illness, hematologic malignancy, bone marrow transplant, and mucositis.

It should be noted that the role of antibiotic selective pressure in promoting enterococcal colonization and infection was recognized prior to the appearance of VRE. Soon after the introduction of broad-spectrum cephalosporins, observational studies reported high rates of enterococcal superinfections in patients treated with these agents [37,38]. Subsequently, case-control studies have shown an association between cephalosporin exposure and enterococcal colonization or infection [39-43]. Antibiotics with activity against anaerobes, including imipenem-cilastatin, metronidazole, and clindamycin, also often have been associated with colonization or infection with vancomycin-susceptible enterococci [44]. Many of the cephalosporins that have been associated with enterococcal infection or colonization, particularly moxalactam and cefoxitin, also have potent activity against anaerobes. The association between antianaerobic antibiotics and enterococcal infection is consistent with previous studies in human volunteers in which administration of antianaerobic antibiotics resulted in overgrowth of enterococci in feces [45].

Table II-4 summarizes the clinical studies that have shown an association between specific classes of antibiotics and VRE colonization or infection. Studies are not included if they demonstrated an association between VRE and antibiotics, but did not implicate specific classes of antibiotics or if the demonstrated antibiotic associations were not statistically significant. Several studies have demonstrated an association between vancomycin exposure and VRE [4,18,36,46-54]. Exposure to cephalosporins or antibiotics with activity against anaerobes has been associated with VRE in multiple studies, similar to the associations observed for vancomycin-susceptible enterococci [35,47,55]. Third-generation cephalosporins have been specifically identified as a risk factor for VRE colonization or infection in several of these studies [46,47,50,51]. Ceftazidime, a third-generation cephalosporin with minimal activity against anaerobes, has been implicated as a risk factor for VRE colonization or infection in one study [48]. In a study we conducted in northeast Ohio, total hospital use of extended-spectrum cephalosporins had a positive (although not statistically significant) correlation with isolation of VRE [28]. A significant positive correlation was shown between the use of ticarcillin-clavulanate and isolation of VRE. These data suggest that some classes of antibiotics may promote colonization and infection with VRE more than others. The association observed between cephalosporins and

Table II-4. Clinical Studies Demonstrating an Association Between Exposure to Certain Classes of Antibiotics and Colonization or Infection With VRE

Reference	Type of Study	Antibiotic	Commentary
Rubin, 1992 [52]	Case-control	Vancomycin	Pediatric oncology patients colonized with VR *E faecium* in stool (8 cases) compared with nonimmunized controls
Karanfil et al, 1992 [53]	Case-control	Vancomycin	Cardiothoracic surgery ICU patients colonized or infected with VR *E faecium* compared with noninfected controls
Livornese et al, 1992 [48]	Case-control	Ceftazidime	ICU patients colonized or infected with VR *E faecium* (duration) compared with uninfected controls (univariate analysis)
Frieden et al, 1993 [24]	Observational	Cephalosporins Vancomycin	VRE clinical isolation was associated with preceding cephalosporin (1st, 2nd, or 3rd generation) and/or vancomycin (IV or PO) treatment
Handwerger et al, 1993 [49]	Case-control	Cephalosporins Aminoglycosides Vancomycin (IV or PO)	ICU patients colonized and/or infected with VRE were compared with noninfected controls (univariate analysis)
Boyle et al, 1993 [54]	Case-control	Vancomycin	Patients with VRE infection compared with controls with infection with vancomycin-susceptible enterococcal infection
Morris et al, 1995 [18]	Case-control	Vancomycin Ciprofloxacin	Surgical ICU and step-down unit patients colonized or infected with VRE were compared with noninfected patients on the same units (multivariate analysis)
Moreno et al, 1995 [50]	Case-control	3rd-generation cephalosporins Vancomycin (IV)	Patients colonized or infected with VanB VR *E faecium* were compared with patients colonized with VSE

(continued)

Table II-4. Clinical Studies Demonstrating an Association Between Exposure to Certain Classes of Antibiotics and Colonization or Infection With VRE (cont)

Reference	Type of Study	Antibiotic	Commentary
Edmond et al, 1995 [35]	Case-control	Antianaerobic antibiotics (metronidazole, clindamycin, imipenem, ampicillin-sulbactam)	Oncology patients with VR *E faecium* bacteremia compared with matched controls from the same ward without VRE bacteremia
Shay et al, 1995 [36]	Case-control	Vancomycin (IV)	Patients with VRE-bloodstream infection compared with patients with VSE-bloodstream infection
Weinstein, 1996 [51]	Prospective Cohort study	3rd-generation cephalosporins Vancomycin Clindamycin	ICU and medical ward patients with nosocomially acquired VRE compared with control patients who did not acquire VRE (univariate analysis)
Tornieporth et al, 1996 [46]	Case-control	3rd-generation cephalosporins Vancomycin	Patients colonized or infected with VanA VR *E faecium* compared patients colonized or infected with VS *E faecium* (multivariate analysis) Hospital 3rd-generation cephalosporin use was: ceftriaxone (51%), ceftazidime (46%), and cefotaxirne (3%)
Beezhold et al, 1997 [47]	Case-control	Vancomycin Metronidazole 3rd-generation cephalosporins Clindamycin	Patients with skin colonization with VRE were compared with control patients not colonized with VRE on skin (univariate analysis)
Lucas et al, 1998 [55]	Case-control	Metronidazole	Patients with VRE bacteremia were compared with patients with VSE bacteremia

Reprinted with permission from Donskey and Rice [44].

antianaerobic antibiotics and vancomycin-susceptible enterococci provide further support for the association between these antibiotics and VRE.

Antibiotics and VRE Colonization in a Mouse Model

An animal model of VRE colonization may provide information that cannot be ascertained by clinical studies. For example, an animal model allows for comparison of the effect of individual antibiotics on VRE colonization. Many case-control studies group similar types of antibiotics together for analysis because the number of patients exposed to individual antibiotics is too small to allow meaningful comparison. Such grouping on the basis of antibiotic class may result in inclusion of individual antibiotics with widely varying levels of biliary excretion and spectra of antimicrobial activity. For example, the cephalosporin cefoperazone has potent antianaerobic activity and significant biliary excretion, but cefepime and ceftazidime have minimal antianaerobic activity and minimal biliary excretion. Similarly, the antianaerobic antibiotics that have been associated with VRE differ significantly in terms of level of biliary excretion and antienterococcal activity. A second advantage of an animal model of VRE colonization is that it allows investigators to control factors such as the size of the VRE inoculum.

We have used a mouse model to study the effect of different subcutaneous antibiotics on the persistence and level of intestinal VRE colonization [56]. Based upon the methods of Whitman et al [57], VRE intestinal colonization in mice was established by performing gastric inoculation of *E faecium* C68, a clinical VanB VRE isolate (vancomycin MIC, 512 mg/mL; ampicillin MIC, 256 mg/mL), in conjunction with administration of oral vancomycin in drinking water. After confirming the presence of high-level VRE colonization, oral vancomycin was discontinued and subcutaneous injection of antibiotics was initiated at 12-hour intervals. Total daily doses of antibiotics were equivalent to the daily dose (per kg) recommended for human adults. Fresh stool specimens were collected at 4- to 5-day intervals, and the level of VRE was quantified by plating on selective media. The level of aerobic and facultative gram-negative rods and total enterococci also were quantified in selected samples.

Prior to beginning administration of subcutaneous antibiotics, all mice were colonized with high levels of VRE (mean = 9.5 $\log_{10}$CFU/g). The effect of subcutaneous antibiotics on persistence and level of colonization is shown in Figures II-3 and II-4. The level of VRE in the stool of normal saline control mice steadily decreased during the 19 days of the experiment, while the level of VRE in the oral vancomycin (positive control) mice remained high. Subcutaneous vancomycin, clindamycin, piperacillin-tazobactam, ticarcillin-clavulanic acid,

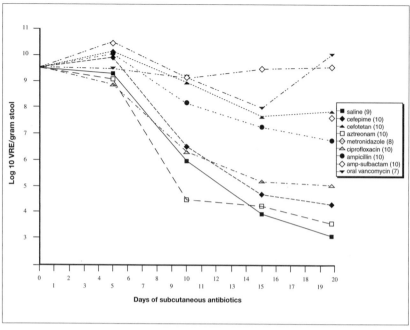

Figures II-3 and II-4. Persistence of VRE intestinal colonization in mice treated with different subcutaneous antibiotics. All mice were colonized with VRE on day 0 (mean 9.5 $\log_{10}$ CFU/g stool). Mice received subcutaneous injections every 12 hours of the antibiotics shown in the Figure legends. Negative control mice received subcutaneous saline and positive controls received oral vancomycin (250 mg/mL) in drinking water. Stool VRE levels were measured by plating diluted samples on selective agar containing vancomycin 6 mg/mL. For comparisons between groups, analysis of variance and linear regression were performed. Pip = piperacillin; tic = ticarcillin. Reprinted with permission from Donskey et al [56].

metronidazole, cefotetan, ampicillin, and ampicillin-sulbactam all promoted persistent high levels of VRE in stool. Subcutaneous ceftriaxone, cefepime, ciprofloxacin, and aztreonam promoted increased VRE levels to a lesser degree or not at all. Thus, in a mouse model, vancomycin and antibiotics with potent activity against anaerobes promoted persistent high levels of stool VRE colonization compared with antibiotics lacking potent activity against anaerobes (including third-generation cephalosporins), which did not. These results suggest that administration of antibiotics with potent activity against anaerobes to patients who are already colonized with VRE may promote persistent high levels

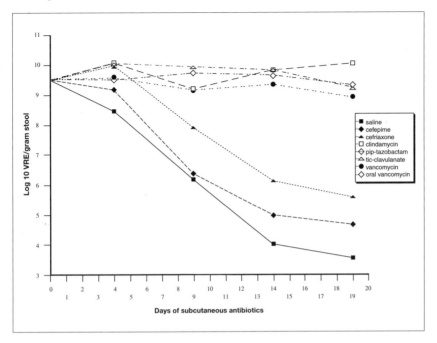

of VRE. Further studies are needed to determine whether these findings are applicable to humans.

Our findings using the mouse model differ from two observations from clinical studies. First, exposure to third-generation cephalosporins with minimal activity against anaerobes (including ceftazidime) has been associated with VRE colonization in multiple studies. Second, Quale et al [58] have reported that restriction of third-generation cephalosporins while increasing the use of piperacillin-tazobactam and ampicillin-sulbactam (antibiotics with potent activity against anaerobes) resulted in a significant decrease in the prevalence of VRE colonization in an outbreak setting. These discrepancies may be due to the fact that this model examined the effect of antibiotics on already established colonization, but not on the initial establishment of colonization. In clinical settings patients may be exposed intermittently to small inocula of VRE. Piperacillin-tazobactam achieves levels in human bile (>1,000 mg/mL) after intravenous injection that are above the MICs of many VRE isolates [59]. Therefore, we have hypothesized that piperacillin-tazobactam treatment may inhibit the establishment of colonization after inoculation of small numbers of VRE. Further studies in mice are planned to test this hypothesis.

Two other investigations have examined the differing effects of antibiotics on VRE colonization of the gastrointestinal tracts of rats and mice. Louie and associates [60] challenged rats with ceftriaxone or piperacillin-tazobactam, then attempted colonization with VRE. Ceftriaxone-treated rats were easily colonized by VRE, piperacillin-tazobactam-treated animals were able to suppress VRE colonization, and antibiotic-free controls were relatively resistant to colonization. In the mouse study, administration of ceftriaxone, ticarcillin-clavulanate, or piperacillin-tazobactam was begun two days prior to colonization with VRE and continued for 16 additional days [61]. The two antibiotics with minimal antienterococcal activity (ceftriaxone and ticarcillin-clavulanate) promoted establishment of high-level VRE colonization that persisted during antibiotic administration, but piperacillin-tazobactam did not. These results suggest that antibiotics may have significantly different influences on the establishment of intestinal colonization with VRE.

Control of Vancomycin Resistance

In 1994, the Centers for Disease Control and Prevention's Hospital Infection Control Practices Advisory Committee (HICPAC) published recommendations for preventing and controlling the spread of vancomycin resistance [62]. This publication stressed the need for a coordinated, multidisciplinary effort requiring participation of the microbiology laboratory, infection control department, pharmacy, housekeeping services, and all personnel who come in direct contact with patients. Specific recommendations were made for surveillance measures to identify patients colonized or infected with VRE, isolation measures to prevent person-to-person transmission of VRE, and prudent use of vancomycin.

Surveillance
The initial recognition of the presence of VRE isolates in a hospital system depends on the ability of the microbiology laboratory to identify vancomycin-resistant clinical strains correctly. For hospitals where VRE have not been detected previously, clinical enterococcal isolates should be screened periodically for vancomycin resistance. Laboratories should be aware that automated susceptibility testing methods may not correctly identify VanB VRE strains with relatively low levels of vancomycin resistance (MICs ranging from 8 to 32 mg/mL) [62]. These strains are correctly identified by agar disk diffusion testing [62].

When VRE are identified in a medical facility, a surveillance system for identification of colonized or infected patients should be instituted, and all clinical enterococcal isolates should be tested for vancomycin resistance [62]. Some form of surveillance for intestinal colonization is recommended because most patients harboring VRE are not detected if only clinical samples are screened. In the Cleveland area, some hospitals screen all stool samples submitted to the microbiology department for the presence of VRE. At one hospital employing this surveillance technique, approximately 90% of all isolates detected represent stool colonization without concurrent clinical isolation of VRE (Robert Salata, personal communication). Additional prevalence surveys for intestinal colonization may be indicated periodically for high-risk patients or units. For detection of intestinal colonization, perirectal cultures have been shown to correlate well with internal rectal swabs [62].

Isolation Measures to Prevent Person-to-Person Transmission

HICPAC recommendations for isolation measures to prevent person-to-person transmission of VRE in all hospitals include:

- Place patients who have evidence of VRE in private rooms or in rooms with other patients who have VRE infection or colonization.
- Wear gloves when entering a VRE-colonized or -infected patient's room and wear a gown if substantial contact with the patient or environment is anticipated.
- Remove gloves and gown before leaving the room and wash with antiseptic soap.
- Dedicate the use of items such as stethoscopes, blood pressure cuffs, and thermometers to a single patient (or group of patients) colonized or infected with VRE.

These isolation measures, in combination with surveillance cultures, have been shown to be effective in eliminating small VRE outbreaks due to dissemination single strains of VRE. Boyce et al [17] reported a hospital outbreak of clonal VanB-type VRE that persisted despite placement of patients with VRE in private rooms and the requirement that all healthcare workers entering these rooms wear gloves. However, when healthcare workers entering the rooms of affected patients were required to wear both gloves and gowns, the outbreak was terminated. These investigators commented that the use of gowns may have reduced the acquisition of environmental VRE by healthcare workers or that requiring gown use may have led to improved compliance with glove use and handwashing.

Infection control measures have not been as effective in the setting of large polyclonal VRE outbreaks [18,28]. Wells et al [63] reported that infection control practices, including isolation measures and surveillance cultures, were not effective in reducing VRE transmission in the setting of a polyclonal outbreak.

Slaughter et al [64] found that use of gloves and gowns was not more effective than use of gloves alone in preventing rectal colonization with VRE in a medical intensive care unit of a hospital experiencing a large polyclonal outbreak. In the Cleveland-area outbreak, we observed that several local hospitals developed significant VRE outbreaks despite institution of infection control measures shortly after VRE initially were isolated [28].

Restriction of Vancomycin Use

The HICPAC guidelines recommend restricting use of vancomycin to settings where its use is clearly indicated [62]. Situations in which the use of vancomycin was considered appropriate or acceptable included treatment of infections in patients with serious β-lactam allergies, treatment of serious infections caused by β-lactam-resistant gram-positive organisms, treatment of *C difficile* colitis that is severe or unresponsive to metronidazole therapy, single-dose surgical prophylaxis of patients at high risk for methicillin-resistant *S aureus* or *S epidermidis*, and occasionally for endocarditis prophylaxis as recommended by the American Heart Association. A number of specific situations in which use of vancomycin was discouraged were listed as well. It should be noted that restriction of oral and intravenous vancomycin did not reduce the prevalence of VRE colonization in one large, polyclonal outbreak, although a relatively low rate of colonization was maintained [18]. Ultimately, restriction of vancomycin is not likely to eradicate VRE outbreaks because other widely used antibiotics also select for growth of multidrug-resistant VRE.

Restriction of Antibiotics Other Than Vancomycin

At this time, few published reports have examined the efficacy of restricting antibiotics other than vancomycin for control of VRE outbreaks. Quale et al [58] altered the antibiotic formulary at a Veterans Affairs hospital by restricting use of third-generation cephalosporins, vancomycin, and clindamycin while increasing use of ampicillin-sulbactam and piperacillin-tazobactam. After 6 months, monthly use of cefotaxime, ceftazidime, vancomycin, and clindamycin had decreased by 84%, 55%, 34%, and 80%, respectively. The point prevalence of fecal colonization with VRE decreased from 47% to 15% ($P < 0.001$), and isolation of VRE from clinical specimens also decreased. These authors concluded that the change in antibiotic use resulted in the decrease in VRE colonization rate, although concurrent control of a *C difficile* outbreak and increased infection control measures may also have played roles.

In a recent prospective cohort study, Montecalvo et al [65] reported that an enhanced infection control strategy that included a program for reducing total antimicrobial use resulted in reduced VRE transmission in an oncology unit compared with standard VRE infection control practices (HICPAC guidelines). Compared with the standard infection control period, use of vancomycin, imipenem-cilastatin, ceftazidime, ciprofloxacin, aztreonam, and gentamicin during the enhanced infection control period was significantly reduced. The incidence of both VRE bloodstream infections and rectal colonization decreased significantly during the enhanced infection control period.

Faced with an outbreak of glycopeptide-resistant enterococci (GRE/VRE) in a hematologic unit, Bradley and colleagues [66] manipulated their antibiotic formulary from empiric use of ceftazidime to empiric use of piperacillin-tazobactam and instituted stringent infection control measures. These maneuvers decreased colonization and infection significantly ($P<0.0001$). In a rechallenge study within the unit, empiric ceftazidime replaced piperacillin/tazobactam in the last phase of the investigation. Within 3 months, the incidence of VRE colonization increased substantially.

These studies lend support to the hypothesis that restriction of antibiotics other than vancomycin may play a role in limiting the spread of VRE. However, the amount of the reduction in the incidence of VRE that can be attributed to changes or reductions in antibiotic use is not clear because other infection control measures were implemented or intensified concurrently. For example, in the study by Montecalvo et al [65], several different classes of antibiotics were restricted simultaneously, which makes it unclear whether restriction of specific antibiotics played a disproportionate role in decreasing the rate of VRE infection and colonization.

Intestinal Decolonization

Eradication of stool carriage of VRE would remove the most important reservoir for spread of these organisms. Several small studies have evaluated the efficacy of using antibiotic therapy for this purpose. Montecalvo et al [67] reported that treatment with oral novobiocin in combination with doxycycline or tetracycline was not effective in eradicating VRE stool carriage. Chia and co-workers [68] treated patients colonized with VRE with oral bacitracin twice daily for 10 days, then collected perirectal swab cultures for VRE at weekly intervals for 3 weeks. They found that 63% (5/8) of patients had negative rectal cultures for VRE for 3 weeks of follow-up, and an additional patient had negative cultures after a second course of treatment. One of these patients subsequently relapsed after receiving antibiotic therapy for another infection. Weinstein et al [69] recently reported findings from a prospective observational cohort study on a renal ward that was designed to assess the effectiveness of 14 days of oral bacitracin plus doxycycline for eradication of VRE colonization. All 15 patients treated with these antibiotics had negative rectal swabs for VRE on day 14 compared with 33% (8/24) of untreated control patients. However, with longer periods of follow-up (from 1 to 4 months after treatment), there was no significant difference in colonization status between the treatment and control groups (60% of treated and 62.5% of untreated control patients carried VRE intermittently or persistently). No significant differences in antibiotic therapy during the follow-up period were observed between the two groups. Quantitative VRE stool cultures revealed that patients treated with bacitracin and doxycycline initially had a 3 $\log_{10}$CFU/g decrease in VRE levels, but the level of VRE subsequently returned to pretreatment levels (mean, 7.8 $\log_{10}$CFU/g).

The data from these studies suggest that oral bacitracin therapy reduces the level of stool VRE during therapy, but the effect is transient, and there is a rapid return to pretreatment levels for many patients. Similar results were reported for VRE-colonized mice treated with oral daptomycin [70]. Based on these studies, it does not appear likely that short courses of antibiotics with activity against VRE will provide a solution to the problem of long-term colonization with VRE.

Conclusion

Based upon current epidemiologic trends, it is likely that VRE will continue to spread and increase in importance as nosocomial pathogens in the United States. It is imperative for the pharmaceutical industry to continue intensive efforts toward developing effective antimicrobial agents to treat patients infected with VRE. Further studies also are needed to optimize the effectiveness of infection control strategies for VRE. Data derived from a mouse model of VRE intestinal colonization and from case-control studies suggest that selective use of antibiotics may be an effective measure to limit the spread of these organisms. Prospective interventional studies to test the effectiveness of this strategy are needed. Finally, further studies of intestinal decolonization will clarify the role of this strategy for controlling the spread of VRE.

References

1. Boyce JM, Mermel LA, Zervos MJ, et al. Controlling vancomycin-resistant enterococci. *Infect Control Hosp Epidemiol.* 1995;16:634-637.
2. Murray BE. The life and times of the enterococcus. *Clin Microbiol Rev.* 1990;3:46-65.
3. Center for Disease Control and Prevention. Nosocomial enterococci resistant to vancomycin-United States, 1989-1993. *MMWR Morbid Mort Week Rep.* 1993;42:597-599.
4. Edmond MB. Multidrug-resistant enterococci and the threat of vancomycin-resistant *Staphylococcus aureus*. In: Wenzel RP, ed. *Prevention and Control of Nosocomial Infections.* 3rd ed.

Baltimore, Md: Williams and Wilkins; 1997:339-355.

5. Murray BE. Vancomycin-resistant enterococci. *Am J Med.* 1997;101:284-293.

6. Emori TG, Gaynes RP. An overview of nosocomial infections, including the role of the micro-biology laboratory. *Clin Microbiol Rev.* 1993;6:428-442.

7. Fontana R, Grossato A, Rossi L, Cheng YR, Satta G. Transition from resistance to hypersuscep-tibility to β-lactam antibiotics associated with loss of a low affinity penicillin-binding protein in a *Streptococcus faecium* mutant highly resistant to penicillin. *Antimicrob Agents Chemother.* 1985;28:678-683.

8. Geraci JE, Martin WJ. Subacute enterococcal endocarditis: clinical, pathologic and therapeutic considerations in 33 patients. *Circulation.* 1954;10:173-194.

9. Jawetz E, Sonne M. Penicillin-streptomycin treatment of enterococcal endocarditis: a reevalu-ation. *N Engl J Med.* 1966;274:710-715.

10. Rice LB, Calderwood SB, Eliopoulos GM, Farber BF, Karchmer AW. Enterococcal endocardi-tis: a comparison of native and prosthetic valve disease. *Rev Infect Dis.* 1991; 13:1-7.

11. Eliopoulos GM, Wennersten C, Zighelboim-Daum S, Reiszner E, Goldmann D, Moellering RC Jr. High-level resistance to gentamicin in clinical isolates of *Streptococcus (Enterococcus) faecium. Antimicrob Agents Chemother.* 1988;32:1528-1532.

12. Carias LL, Rudin SD, Donskey CJ, Rice LB. Genetic linkage and co-transfer of a novel, *vanB-*encoding transposon (Tn*5382*) and a low-affinity penicillin-binding protein 5 gene in a clinical vancomycin-resistant *Enterococcus faecium* isolate. *J Bacteriol.* 1998;180:4426-4434.

13. Arthur M, Reynolds P, Courvalin P. Glycopeptide resistance in enterococci. *Trends Microbiol.* 1996;4:401-407.

14. Rice LB, Shlaes DM. Vancomycin resistance in the enterococcus: relevance in pediatrics. *Pediatr Clin North Am.* 1995;42:601-617.

15. Perichon B, Reynolds P, Courvalin P. VanD-type glycopeptide-resistant *Enterococcus faecium* BM4339. *Antimicrob Agents Chemother.* 1997;41:2016-2018.

16. Fines M, Perichon B, Reynolds P, Sahm DF, Courvalin P. VanE, a new type of acquired glyco-peptide resistance in *E. faecalis* BM4405. *Antimicrob Agents Chemother.* 1999;43:2161-2164.

17. Boyce JM, Opal SM, Chow JW, et al. Outbreak of multidrug-resistant *Enterococcus faecium* with transferable *vanB* class vancomycin resistance. *J Clin Microbiol.* 1994;32:1148-1153.

18. Morris JG, Shay DK, Hebden JN, et al. Enterococci resistant to multiple antimicrobial agents, including vancomycin: establishment of endemicity in a university medical center. *Ann Intern Med.* 1995;123:250-259.

19. Arthur M, Molinas C, Depardieu F, Courvalin P. Characterization of Tn*1546,* a Tn*3*-related transposon conferring glycopeptide resistance by synthesis of depsipeptide peptidoglycan pre-cursors in *Enterococcus faecium* BM4147. *J Bacteriol.* 1993;175:117-127.

20. Quintiliani R Jr, Courvalin P. Characterization of Tn*1547,* a composite transposon flanked by the IS*16* and IS*256*-like elements, that confers vancomycin resistance in *Enterococcus faecium* BM4281. *Gene.* 1996;172:1-8.

21. Rice LB, Carias LL, Donskey CJ, Rudin SD. Transferable, plasmid-mediated VanB-type glyco-peptide resistance in *Enterococcus faecium. Antimicrob Agents Chemother.* 1998;42:963-964.

22. Rice LB. The theoretical origin of vancomycin-resistant enterococci. *Clin Microbiol Newslet-ter.* 1995;17:189-192.

23. Leclerq R, Derlot E, Duval J, Courvalin P. Plasmid-mediated resistance to vancomycin and teicoplanin in *Enterococcus faecium. N Engl J Med.* 1988;319:157-161.

24. Frieden TR, Munsiff SS, Lowe DE, et al. Emergence of vancomycin resistant enterococci in

New York City. *Lancet.* 1993;342:76-79.

25. Trick WE, Kuehnert MJ, Quirk SB, et al. Regional dissemination of vancomycin-resistant enterococci resulting from interfacility transfer of colonized patients. *J Infect Dis.* 1999;180:391-396.

26. Schwalbe RS, McIntosh AC, Qaiyumi S, Johnson JA, Morris JG. Isolation of vancomycin-resistant enterococci from animal feed in USA. *Lancet.* 1999;353:722.

27. Chow JW, Kuritza A, Shlaes DM, Green M, Sahm DF, Zervos MJ. Clonal spread of vancomycin resistant *Enterococcus faecium* between patients in three hospitals in two states. *J Clin Microbiol.* 1993;31:1609-1611.

28. Donskey CJ, Schreiber JR, Jacobs MR, et al. A polyclonal outbreak of predominantly VanB vancomycin-resistant enterococci in Northeast Ohio. *Clin Infect Dis.* 1999;29:573-579.

29. Klare I, Badstubner D, Konstabel C, Bohme G, Claus H, Witte W. Decreased incidence of VanA-type vancomycin-resistant enterococci isolated from poultry meat and from fecal samples of humans in the community after discontinuation of avoparcin usage in animal husbandry. *Microbial Drug Resist.* 1999;5:45-51.

30. van der Auwera P, Pensart N, Korten V, Murray BE, Leclercq R. Influence of oral glycopeptides on the fecal flora of human volunteers: selection of highly glycopeptide-resistant enterococci. *J Infect Dis.* 1996;173:1129-1136.

31. Klare I, Heier H, Claus H, Reissbrodt R, Witte W. *vanA*-mediated high-level glycopeptide resistance in *Enterococcus faecium* from animal husbandry. *FEMS Microbiol Letters.* 1995;125:165-172.

32. van den Bogaard AE, Jensen LB, Stobberingh EE. Vancomycin-resistant enterococci in turkeys and farmers. *N Engl J Med.* 1997;337:1558-1559.

33. Poyart C, Pierre C, Quiesne G, Pron B, Berche P, Trieu-Cuot P. Emergence of vancomycin resistance in the genus *Streptococcus:* characterization of a *vanB* transferable determinant in *Streptococcus bovis. Antimicrob Agents Chemother.* 1997;41:24-29.

34. Montecalvo MA, de Lencastre H, Carraher M, et al. Natural history of colonization with vancomycin-resistant *Enterococcus faecium. Infect Control Hosp Epidemiol.* 1995;16:680-685.

35. Edmond MB, Ober JF, Weinbaum DL, et al. Vancomycin-resistant *Enterococcus faecium* bacteremia: risk factors for infection. *Clin Infect Dis.* 1995;20:1126-1133.

36. Shay DK, Maloney SA, Montecalvo M, et al. Epidemiology and mortality risk of vancomycin-resistant enterococcal bloodstream infections. *J Infect Dis.* 1995;172:993-1000.

37. Yu V. Enterococcal superinfection and colonization after therapy with moxalactam, a new broad-spectrum antibiotic. *Ann Intern Med.* 1981;94:784-785.

38. Moellering RC Jr. Enterococcal infections in patients treated with moxalactam. *Rev Infect Dis.* 1982;4(suppl):S708-S711.

39. Chirurgi VA, Oster SE, Goldberg AA, McCabe RE. Nosocomial acquisition of β-lactamase-negative, ampicillin-resistant enterococcus. *Arch Intern Med.* 1992;152:1457-1461.

40. Noskin GA, Till M, Patterson BK, Clarke JT, Warren JR. High-level gentamicin resistance in *Enterococcus faecalis* bacteremia. *J Infect Dis.* 1991;164:212-215.

41. Pallares R, Pujol M, Pena C, Ariza J, Martin R, Gudiol F. Cephalosporins as a risk factor for nosocomial *Enterococcus faecalis* bacteremia. *Arch Intern Med.* 1993;153:1581-1586.

42. Weigelt JA, Easley SM, Thal ER, Palmer LD, Newman VS. Abdominal surgical wound infection is lowered with improved perioperative *Enterococcus* and *Bacteroides* therapy. *J Trauma.* 1993;34:579-585.

43. Suppola JP, Volin L, Valtonen VV, Vaara M. Overgrowth of *Enterococcus faecium* in the feces

of patients with hematologic malignancies. *Clin Infect Dis.* 1996;23:694-697.

44. Donskey CJ, Rice LB. The influence of antibiotics on spread of vancomycin-resistant entero-cocci: the potential role of selective use of antibiotics as a control measure. *Clin Microbiol Newsletter.* 1999;21:57-65.

45. Vollaard EJ, Clasener HAL. Colonization resistance. *Antimicrob Agents Chemother.* 1994;38:409-414.

46. Tornieporth NG, Roberts RB, John J, Hafner A, Riley LW. Risk factors associated with van-comycin-resistant *Enterococcus faecium* infection or colonization in 145 matched case patients and control patients. *Clin Infect Dis.* 1996;23:767-772.

47. Beezhold DW, Slaughter S, Hayden MK, et al. Skin colonization with vancomycin-resistant enterococci among hospitalized patients with bacteremia. *Clin Infect Dis.* 1997;24:704-706.

48. Livornese LLJ, Dias S, Samel C. Hospital-acquired infection with vancomycin-resistant *Enterococcus faecium* transmitted by electronic thermometers. *Ann Intern Med.* 1992;117:112-116.

49. Handwerger S, Raucher B, Altarec D, et al. Nosocomial outbreak due to *Enterococcus faecium* highly resistant to vancomycin, penicillin and gentamicin. *Clin Infect Dis.* 1993;16:750-755.

50. Moreno F, Crisp C, Jorgensen JH, Patterson JE. The clinical and molecular epidemiology of bacteremias at a university hospital caused by pneumococci not susceptible to penicillin. *J Infect Dis.* 1995;172:427-432.

51. Weinstein JW. Resistant enterococci: a prospective study of prevalence, incidence, and factors associated with colonization in a university hospital. *Infect Control Hosp Epidemiol.* 1996;17:36-41.

52. Rubin LG. Vancomycin-resistant *Enterococcus faecium* in hospitalized children. *Infect Control Hosp Epidemiol.* 1992;13:700-705.

53. Karanfil LV, Murphy M, Josephson A, et al. A cluster of vancomycin-resistant *Enterococcus faecium* in an intensive care unit. *Infect Control Hosp Epidemiol.* 1992;13:195-200.

54. Boyle JF, Soumakis SA, Rendo A, et al. Epidemiologic analysis and genotypic characterization of a nosocomial outbreak of vancomycin-resistant enterococci. *J Clin Microbiol.* 1993;31:1280-1285.

55. Lucas GM, Lechtzin N, Puryear DW, Yau LL, Flexner CW, Moore RD. Vancomycin-resistant and vancomycin-susceptible enterococcal bacteremia: comparison of clinical features and out-comes. *Clin Infect Dis.* 1998;26:1127-1133.

56. Donskey CJ, Hanrahan JA, Hutton RA, Rice LB. Effect of parenteral antibiotic administration on persistence of vancomycin-resistant Enterococcus faecium in the mouse gastrointestinal tract. *J Infect Dis.* 1999;180:384-390.

57. Whitman MS, Pitsakis PG, DeJesus E, Osborne AJ, Levison ME, Johnson CC. Gastrointestinal tract colonization with vancomycin-resistant *Enterococcus faecium* in an animal model. *Antimicrob Agents Chemother.* 1996;40:1526-1530.

58. Quale J, Landman D, Saurina G, Atwood E, DiTore V, Patel K. Manipulation of a hospital anti-microbial formulary to control an outbreak of vancomycin-resistant enterococci. *Clin Infect Dis.* 1996;23:1020-1025.

59. Taylor EW, Poxon V, Alexander-Williams J, Jackson D. Biliary excretion of piperacillin. *J Int Med Res.* 1983;11:28-31.

60. Louie T, Krulicki W, Mason A, Louie A. Differential effect of piperacillin/tazobactam compared to ceftriaxone on vancomycin-resistant enterococcal (VRE) colonization during quantitative intestinal challenge. Presented at the International Congress on Chemotherapy. Birmingham,

England; 1999.

61. Donskey CJ, Hanrahan JA, Hutton RA, Rice LB. Effect of parenteral antibiotic administration on establishment of colonization with vancomycin-*resistant Enterococcus faecium* in the mouse gastrointestinal tract. Presented at the 37th Annual Infectious Diseases Society of America Meeting. Philadelphia, Pennsylvania; 1999. Abstract 450.

62. Centers for Disease Control and Prevention. Preventing the spread of vancomycin resistance - report from the Hospital Infection Control Practices Advisory Committee. *Federal Register.* 1994;59:25758-25763.

63. Wells CL, Juni BA, Cameron SB, et al. Stool carriage, clinical isolation, and mortality during an outbreak of vancomycin-resistant enterococci in hospitalized medical and/or surgical patients. *Clin Infect Dis.* 1995;21:45-50.

64. Slaughter S, Hayden MK, Nathan C, et al. A comparison of the effect of universal use of gloves and gowns with that of glove use alone on acquisition of vancomycin-resistant enterococci in a medical intensive care unit. *Ann Intern Med.* 1996;125:448-456.

65. Montecalvo MA, Jarvis WR, Uman J, et al. Infection-control measures reduce transmission of vancomycin-resistant enterococci in an endemic setting. *Ann Intern Med.* 1999;99:269-272.

66. Bradley SJ, Wilson ALT, Allen MC, Sher HA, Goldstone AH, Scott GM. The control of hyper-endemic glycopeptide-resistant *Enterococcus* spp. on a haematology unit by changing antibiotic usage. *J Antimicrob Chemother.* 1999;43:261-266.

67. Montecalvo MA, Horowitz H, Wormser GP, Seiter K, Carbonaro CA. Effect of novobiocin-containing antimicrobial regimens on infection and colonization with vancomycin-resistant *Enterococcus faecium. Antimicrob Agents Chemother.* 1995;39:794.

68. Chia JKS, Nakate MM, Park SS, Lewis RP, McKee B. Use of bacitracin therapy for infection due to vancomycin-resistant *Enterococcus faecium. Clin Infect Dis.* 1995;21:1520.

69. Weinstein MR, Dedier H, Brunton J, Campbell I, Conly JM. Lack of efficacy of oral bacitracin plus doxycycline for the eradication of stool colonization with vancomycin-resistant *Enterococcus faecium. Clin Infect Dis.* 1999;29:361-366.

70. Li T, Zhang X, Oliver N, Andrew T, Silverman J, Tally FP. Effect of oral daptomycin on vancomycin-resistant *Enterococcus faecium* gastrointestinal tract colonization in antibiotic-treated mice. Presented at Infectious Diseases Society of America. Denver, Colorado; 1999.

Curtis J. Donskey, MD, Louis B. Rice, MD, Medical Services and Division of Infectious Diseases, Louis Stokes Cleveland VA Medical Center and Case Western Reserve University School of Medicine, Cleveland, Ohio, USA.

III. Problems in Gram-negative Resistance: Extended-spectrum Beta-lactamases

Jan. E. Patterson

Introduction

The first reports of extended-spectrum beta-lactamases (ESBLs) in gram-negative bacilli came from Europe [1,2] and were followed quickly by reports in the United States [3,4]. This type of antimicrobial resistance is now recognized worldwide [5-7]. Although ESBLs are found most frequently in *Klebsiella pneumoniae*, the elements conferring this type of resistance are transferable to other genera, including *Escherichia coli* and others [8]. These pathogens often occur in an outbreak setting and pose a therapeutic dilemma due to resistance to multiple antimicrobials. ESBL-producing *K pneumoniae* isolates also have a propensity for spread by clonal strain transmission from patient to patient, thereby posing an infection control dilemma. Further, ESBL-producing *K pneumoniae* isolates have emerged as polyclonal strains due to dissemination of genetic elements among distinct strains and even distinct genera of gram-negative bacilli. Control interventions for these organisms involve choosing effective therapy for infected patients and instituting infection control and antibiotic utilization measures.

ESBLs

ESBLs are those beta-lactamases that hydrolyze extended-spectrum cephalosporins that have an oxyimino side chain, including ceftazidime, ceftriaxone, cefotaxime, and the oxyimino-monobactam aztreonam. The ESBLs derive from common plasmid-mediated enzyme families of TEM, SHV, and OXA (Table III-

1) [8-10]. Currently, there are at least 61 TEM ESBLs, 12 SHV ESBLs, and 6 ESBLs in the OXA family [13]. The number of identified ESBLs is growing so rapidly that a Web site tracks the number and properties delineating these enzymes [14].

The enzymes have one or more amino acid substitutions that result in an altered configuration and altered active site such that the substrate spectrum is increased. The isoelectric point of the enzyme may also shift as a result of the change. Most enzymes have the greatest hydrolytic activity against ceftazidime and aztreonam followed by cefotaxime, although the opposite holds true for SHV ESBLs and for TEM enzymes with a serine substitution for glycine at the 238 position (G238S) [15]. Enzymes that have single amino acid changes, as in TEM-12, which has serine substituted for arginine at position 164 (R164S), have weaker hydrolytic activity for the oxyimino-beta-lactams and lower MICs to these agents (Table III-1) [13]. TEM-10 is created by an additional substitution of lysine instead of glutamate at position 240. In TEM-26, this substitution occurs at position 104, and the hydrolytic activity for ceftazidime and aztreonam is significantly enhanced. The molecular mechanism for these changes is that the substitutions at positions 104 or 240 increase affinity for ceftazidime by creating an electrostatic bond, while the R164S mutations open the active site of the enzyme to accommodate the large 1-carboxy-1-methylethoxyimino side chain of ceftazidime [16].

In vitro, ESBLs are characteristically susceptible to the beta-lactamase inhibitors clavulanic acid, sulbactam, and tazobactam, and this property is used for in vitro confirmation of the presence of ESBLs. However, beta-lactamase inhibitor combinations do not have consistent therapeutic efficacy for these organisms.

Problems in ESBL Detection

Detection of in vitro resistance is but one of the clinical dilemmas with ESBL-producing gram-negative bacilli. Although these organisms may appear susceptible at a standard inoculum of 10^5, they have highly elevated minimum inhibitory concentrations (MICs) at higher inoculums of 10^7 or 10^8 [15,17]. This inoculum is seen with the third-generation cephalosporins cefotaxime, ceftriaxone, and ceftazidime as well as the "fourth"-generation cephalosporin cefipime. The National Committee on Clinical Laboratory Standards (NCCLS) has recommended detection of ESBLs in *K pneumoniae* and *E coli* by recognizing decreased susceptibility to ceftazidime, cefotaxime, ceftriaxone, or aztreonam that may not reach the previously established thresholds for resistance [18]. A strain

Table III-1. Properties of Extended-spectrum Beta-lactamases

Beta-lactamase	Substitution[†]	pI	MIC*					
			ATM	CAZ	CRO	CTX	CTT	FOX
TEM-1	None	5.4	0.12	0.12	≤0.06	0.06	≤0.25	≤2
TEM-10	R164S, E240K	5.6	16	128	0.5	1	0.25	≤2
TEM-12	R164S	5.25	0.5	3	0.12	0.12	0.12	4
TEM-26	E104K, R164S	5.6	64	256	1	2	0.25	≤2
SHV-1	None	7.6	0.12	0.5	≤0.06	0.06	≤0.25	≤2
SHV-4	R205L, G238S, E240K	7.8	256	128	8	8	0.25	≤2
SHV-5	G238S, E240K	8.2	128	64	4	2	0.12	≤2
MIR-1	Not known	8.4	16	16	16	16	64	256

*Minimum inhibitory concentrations (MICs) were performed by agar dilution on Mueller-Hinton medium with an inoculum of 10^4 organisms per spot [11].

[†]In the substitution designation, the amino acid present in the parental sequence is listed first, then the residue number according to Ambler et al [11], and then the amino acid present in the mutant.

pI=isoelectric point; ATM=aztreonam; CAZ=ceftazidime; CRO=ceftriaxone; CTX=cefotaxime; CTT=cefotetan; FOX=cefoxitin; E=glutamic acid; G=glycine; K=lysine; L=leucine; R=arginine; S=serine.

Adapted from Jacoby GA [13].

of *K pneumoniae* or *E coli* that has an MIC of ≥2 mg/mL to one of these antimicrobials probably produces an ESBL. Recommendations for interpretation of Kirby-Bauer disk zone diameters have also been revised, using diameters of ≤22 mm for ceftazidime, ≤25 mm for ceftriaxone, and ≤27 mm for cefotaxime or aztreonam. The most sensitive substrate for detection of ESBL in *K pneumoniae*, however, may be cefpodoxime, when tested by MIC or disk diffusion using standard breakpoints [18]. This agent is less specific when testing with *E coli*.

The NCCLS recommends that isolates found to produce ESBL be considered resistant to all penicillins, cephalosporins, and aztreonam, regardless of in vitro results. Once an ESBL is suspected, it may be confirmed by several methods, including the double-disk approximation test, three-dimensional agar test, investigational Vitek® ESBL card, or Etest® ESBL strip [17-19]. These tests will distinguish AmpC-type enzymes (which are not inhibited by beta-lactamase inhibitors) from the ESBL enzymes.

Prevalence and Risk Factors for ESBLs

The prevalence of ESBLs is probably underestimated based on a survey by the NCCLS [20]. The Centers for Disease Control and Prevention have noted a dramatic increase in the prevalence of ESBL-producing isolates among *K pneumoniae* in the National Nosocomial Infection Surveillance (NNIS) study, particularly in intensive care units [21-23]. Estimates of ESBL-producing isolates among *K pneumoniae* range from 10.7% in the United States to 20% in a global surveillance program [21, Ron Jones, personal communication, SENTRY Antimicrobial Surveillance Program, 1997 and 1998, University of Iowa].

Case-control studies from multiple outbreaks of ESBL-producing organisms have evaluated risk factors for colonization or infection. Reported risk factors include: presence of intravascular catheters (central venous catheter, arterial catheter), emergency intra-abdominal surgery, gastrostomy or jejunostomy tube, gastrointestinal colonization, length of hospital or intensive care unit stay, prior antibiotics (including third-generation cephalosporins), prior nursing home stay, severity of illness, presence of a urinary catheter, and ventilator assistance (Table III-2) [5,24-29]. Clearly, these organisms affect severely ill patients in the intensive care unit setting as well as chronically debilitated patients in the long-term care setting.

Table III-2. Risk Factors for Infection or Colonization With Extended-spectrum Beta-lactamase-producing *Enterobacteriaceae* in Case-Control Studies

Intravascular devices	Gastrointestinal colonization
Arterial catheter	Previous antibiotics
Central venous catheter	Previous exposure to ceftazidime
Gastrostomy or jejunostomy tube	or aztreonam
Urinary catheter	Severity of illness
Prior nursing home residence	Ventilatory assistance
Low birthweight	Length of intensive care unit stay
Emergency abdominal surgery	Length of hospital stay

Data from [5,24-28]. Adapted from Jacoby GA [13].

The Therapeutic Dilemma: An Overview

Due to the broad spectrum of the beta-lactamase produced by these organisms, ESBL-producing *Enterobacteriaceae* are typically resistant to beta-lactam antibiotics, including broad-spectrum cephalosporins, aztreonam, and extended-spectrum penicillins. Other resistance determinants, including trimethoprim/sulfamethoxazole and aminoglycosides, especially gentamicin, are often cotransferred on a resistance plasmid, resulting in multiple drug resistance [30,31]. Some ESBL-producing strains are susceptible to the cephamycins, cefoxitin, and cefotetan. However, there are increasing reports of coexisting AmpC-type beta-lactamases that are resistant to the cephamycins [20,32] and emergence of porin-deficient mutants during therapy with a cephamycin [33].

The fluoroquinolones may be useful for therapy when the organisms are susceptible to these agents, but many ESBL-producing gram-negative isolates are also resistant to the fluoroquinolones [31]. Although fluoroquinolone resistance was thought previously to be chromosomally mediated, there is now a report of plasmid-mediated fluoroquinolone resistance in *K pneumoniae* [34]. Fluoroquinolone resistance in ESBL-producing gram-negative bacilli is likely to be multifactorial and may be associated with the exposure of these organisms to antibiotic selection pressure in the intensive care unit and/or the long-term care unit.

The Problem with Cephalosporins
One of the problems with cephalosporins and ESBL producers is detecting

in vitro resistance [17]. As discussed previously, these organisms may appear susceptible at a standard inoculum of 10^5, but at higher inoculums of 10^7 or 10^8 they have elevated MICs, indicating resistance. This inoculum effect is seen with the third-generation cephalosporins such as ceftazidime, cefotaxime, and ceftriaxone [34]. Although the more recently released "fourth"-generation cephalosporin cefepime is more resistant to ESBL hydrolysis, susceptibilities decrease as the inoculum increases [13]. One study has documented less of an in vitro inoculum effect with the oral cephalosporin ceftibuten, but this phenomenon was shown only for organisms with TEM ESBLs and not for SHV ESBLs, which are increasing in prevalence [35]. The inoculum effect has been demonstrated to be significant and/or dose-dependent in most in vivo studies [36,37].

Reports of experience using cephalosporins for infections caused by ESBL-producing organisms suggest the clinical significance of the in vitro inoculum effect. One of the early reports was from Rice et al [29] during an outbreak at a chronic care facility in Massachusetts. Of 29 patients who had evidence of the organism, 14 had infections. These 14 were treated with a variety of agents, including cefotaxime, amikacin, trimethoprim/sulfamethoxazole, and ciprofloxacin, and each responded. However, the four patients who received cefotaxime were not bacteremic. One of the larger experiences is reported by Meyer et al [38], who documented a 2-year outbreak of ESBL-producing *K pneumoniae* that involved 155 colonized or infected patients. Therapy and outcome were evaluated in 48 patients who had infection. Thirteen patients who had invasive infection and did not receive therapy directed against ESBLs died. Two patients who had nonbacteremic bacteriuria responded to cephalosporins. Naumovski et al [39] reported experience with ESBL-producing *K pneumoniae* bacteremia in four oncology patients. Two who received only ceftazidime died; two who received a combination of ceftazidime and tobramycin survived. Karas et al [40] reported another ESBL *K pneumoniae* bacteremia that was treated unsuccessfully with cefotaxime.

More recently, Paterson and associates [5] have presented a global study of *K pneumoniae* bacteremia in more than 200 patients from seven hospitals on six continents. The 15% of patients who had ESBL isolates were compared with 85% of patients who had non-ESBL isolates. A total of 84% of ESBL patients had hospital-acquired bacteremias compared with 43% of those who had non-ESBL bacteremia. Third-generation cephalosporins had been administered recently to 31% of ESBL patients, but only 3% of non-ESBL patients. Imipenem use and piperacillin/tazobactam use were not associated with ESBL infections. The crude mortality of the patients who had ESBL bacteremia was 46% compared with 34% in the non-ESBL group. Nonintensive care unit mortality was also higher among ESBL patients (44% versus 28%). Among bacteremic patients who had ESBLs and received initial empiric therapy to which the organism was resistant, mortality was 75%. Mortality was 28% among those who received initial empiric therapy to which the organism was susceptible.

The Problem with Cephamycins

Although the TEM and SHV ESBLs do not effectively hydrolyze the cephamycins cefoxitin and cefotetan, some ESBL-producing strains have also acquired a plasmid-mediated *ampC* gene. This genetic element mediates an AmpC-type beta-lactamase, a group 1 beta-lactamase that effectively hydrolyzes the cephamycins. Since initial reports of this mechanism as a plasmid-mediated trait, there have been numerous reports from many European and Asian countries as well as multiple hospitals in the United States [6,20,32,41,42].

Another problem with the cephamycins is the emergence of resistant isolates during therapy with these agents [43]. This was reported by Martinez-Martinez et al [33] in a patient receiving cefotetan for an ESBL-producing *K pneumoniae* infection. A mutant was selected in vivo in this patient that had acquired resistance to cefotetan. Further study in the laboratory documented that the isolate that became resistant during cefotetan therapy was a porin-deficient mutant, which was the probable explanation for the emergence of cephamycin resistance. In addition, this mutant had slightly higher MICs to fluoroquinolones.

The Problem with Beta-lactamase Inhibitor Combinations

Because the ESBLs are group 2 beta-lactamases that are usually susceptible to beta-lactamase inhibitors such as clavulanic acid, sulbactam, or tazobactam, use of combination antibiotics containing these agents has been considered. However, the ESBL strains often contain a coexisting AmpC-type enzyme, which is a group 1 beta-lactamase. Beta-lactamase inhibitor combinations are not reliably effective against these beta-lactamases. Porin-deficient mutants have also been reported, which limit access of these agents to their site of action. In addition, Rice et al [36] have demonstrated that a combination of TEM and SHV enzymes, which is frequently present in these organisms, can limit both in vitro and in vivo activity. In vivo studies of cefotaxime/clavulanate and piperacillin/tazobactam combinations have yielded mixed results that appear to be highly dependent on dosing of the agent and type of enzymes present [36,37]. A study of bactericidal activity using time-kill curves demonstrated equivalent bactericidal activity with a cefotaxime + amoxicillin/clavulanate +/- amikacin regimen compared to imipenem +/- amikacin [44]. However, the logistics of the former regimen must be considered as well as the variables of dosing and type of enzymes present in individual strains. Thus, detection of an ESBL does not imply susceptibility to beta-lactamase inhibitor combinations, and another agent should be chosen for therapy of a serious infection.

The Problem with Fluoroquinolones

Fluoroquinolone resistance is often present in ESBL-producing organisms [15,30]. This may be due in part to the risk factors for antimicrobial resistance, including previous exposure to antimicrobials, that are present in hospitalized patients who acquire these strains [15]. A survey of a group of ESBL isolates from the United States documented that 40% were resistant to both gentamicin and ciprofloxacin, which the authors suggested may be related to a selected decrease in membrane permeability [30]. Of concern is the report by Martinez-Martinez et al [32] documenting the emergence of a porin-deficient mutant with elevated MICs to the fluoroquinolones.

Fluoroquinolone resistance almost invariably has been a chromosomally mediated trait when studied in the past, but a recent report has documented transferable fluoroquinolone resistance in *K pneumoniae* on a plasmid that also encodes an AmpC-type beta-lactamase. This suggests the potential for further spread of fluoroquinolone resistance in these problematic organisms. There are reports of satisfactory therapy with the fluoroquinolones when isolates are susceptible [29,41].

The Problem with Aminoglycosides

As discussed previously, many of these organisms are already gentamicin-resistant due to cotransfer of aminoglycoside resistance on a resistance plasmid. Other aminoglycoside resistance, such as amikacin resistance, also may be more common in ESBL-producing isolates [38]. A practical issue is the concern for nephrotoxicity in the severely ill patients who usually acquire these strains, making aminoglycoside therapy less than desirable as an alternative.

The Problem with Carbapenems

At present, imipenem appears to be the best alternative for therapy of serious infections due to ESBL-producing *Enterobacteriacae*. These compounds are highly stable to beta-lactamase hydrolysis [45]. Plasmid-mediated carbapenemases have been reported from Japan [46], but are currently quite rare. Chromosomally mediated carbapenemases are not uncommon. Porin penetration is facilitated by the small molecular size and zwitterionic structure of the carbapenems.

Clinical experience reported to date has been best with these agents. In the large outbreak reported by Meyer et al [38] in which therapy and outcome was reviewed in 48 patients, those who received imipenem had the most favorable outcome. In the recent data presented by Paterson and associates [5] from a multicenter study, patients who had bacteremia caused by ESBL *K pneumoniae* and who received imipenem as therapy had a mortality of 23% compared with 42% when another active antibiotic was used.

Carbapenem therapy, however, is not without complications, including the potential for emergence of resistant organisms. In one outbreak, as imipenem use increased, a strain of *Acinetobacter baumannii* that was resistant to multiple antibiotics, including imipenem, became prevalent [38]. Others have reported cefoxitin and imipenem resistance in *K pneumoniae* isolates that possessed both the AmpC-type beta-lactamase and loss of an outer membrane protein [42]. Organisms that have intrinsic resistance to impenem, such as *Stenotrophomonas maltophilia* and vancomycin-resistant *Enterococcus faecium,* also are of concern. In addition, imipenem lowers the seizure threshold, a particular concern for patients who have renal insufficiency. Although meropenem may have less propensity for this adverse effect, both meropenem and carbapenem are relatively expensive on most hospital formularies, raising another practical concern for their widespread use.

Molecular Epidemiology of ESBL Outbreaks and Implications for Control Measures

The microbiology and molecular epidemiology of ESBL outbreaks indicate that the mechanism of this problem may be due to clonal strain dissemination, plasmid dissemination and selection among polyclonal strains, or both mechanisms (Table III-3).

Diversity of Outbreaks
Rice et al [29] reported one of the early ESBL outbreaks in the United States at a chronic care facility in Youville, Massachusetts. ESBLs were documented among five different genera: *K pneumoniae* (most isolates), *Enterobacter cloacae, E aerogenes, Citrobacter diversus, E coli,* and *Serratia marcescens.* Resistance plasmid dissemination was suggested as the mechanism. Bingen et al [47] from France used molecular epidemiologic techniques to study a complex ESBL *K pneumoniae* outbreak in which several strains with different plasmid contents were spread from patient to patient, sporadic cases of distinct strains occurred, and plasmid dissemination between two distinct strains was documented. Resistance plasmid dissemination among distinct *K pneumoniae* strains and a strain

Table III-3. Molecular Epidemiology of Extended-spectrum Beta-lactamase Outbreaks: Representative Examples of Polyclonal and Clonal Strain Outbreaks

Authors	Country	Predominant Enzyme
Polyclonal Strain Outbreaks		
Rice et al [29]	US	TEM-12, TEM-26
Bingen et al [47]	France	ND
Branger et al [51]	France	TEM-3, SHV-2
Prodinger et al [48]	Austria	SHV-5
Schiappa et al [25]	US	TEM-10
Sader et al [30]	US	ND
Marchese et al [50]	Italy	SHV-5
Rasmussen et al [52]	US	TEM-10
Clonal Strain Outbreaks		
Bauernfeind et al [54]	Germany	SHV-5
French et al [56]	US	SHV-5
Monnet et al [57]	US	ND
Arlet et al [58]	France	SHV-4
Rice et al [60]	US	TEM-6
Decre et al [67]	France	SHV-4
Urban et al [61]	US	TEM-26

US=United States; ND=not determined

of *K oxytoca* and *E coli* was a predominant mechanism of spread in an Austrian hospital [48]. A polyclonal ESBL outbreak was reported by Schiappa et al [25] in Chicago that involved eight different strains of *K pneumoniae* and six different strains of *E coli*. There were some instances of cross-transmission of specific strains by temporal and geographic clustering. In an examination of isolates from 43 United States medical centers in 26 states, some intrahospital and inter-hospital transmission was documented, but there was extensive strain diversity [30]. French and Italian investigators determined that several clones in their hospitals were involved in cross-transmission or sporadic occurrences of infection [49,50]. The polyclonal nature of these outbreaks suggest the importance of factors other than clonal strain transmission, including antibiotic selection pressure on resistance plasmid dissemination among distinct clones and genetic mutation.

Branger et al [51] documented five nosocomial outbreaks in three separate hospital wards in France involving four separate strains. They suggested that the emergence of the TEM-3 ESBL in France has been primarily by plasmid dissemination, but emergence of SHV-4 in France has been primarily due to clonal strain dissemination.

There are numerous instances of clonal strain transmission being the primary mechanism for ESBL outbreaks [32, 53-56], including outbreaks involving multiple hospitals [57,58]. Thus, patient-to-patient cross-transmission of strains remains an important mechanism for the emergence of ESBLs.

Isolation Precautions

Infection control isolation precautions involving the use of barriers (gloves, gowns) for contact with infected patients or their immediate environment have been associated with decreased spread of ESBL-producing organisms [38,47,49]. Current Centers for Disease Control and Prevention guidelines recommend Contact Precautions for the control of multidrug-resistant organisms, such as ESBL-producing gram-negative bacilli [59]. Such precautions involve the use of gloves and gowns for contact with patients or their immediate environment. Antisepsis is also important, and handwashing is recommended after removal of gloves. In addition, because interhospital transfer has been documented, notification by institutions when transferring patients who are infected with multidrug-resistant organisms may help to limit spread [57].

Antibiotic Usage Patterns

Although such traditional infection control measures are important, the complex nature of ESBL outbreaks necessitates consideration of other control measures involving antibiotic use. Antibiotic use patterns, in particular the widespread use of ceftazidime, have been associated with the emergence of ESBLs [29,38,58,60-63]. A decrease in ceftazidime use has been associated with control of ESBL emergence in several instances [29,38,60]. Perhaps one of the best examples of this is the report from the Cleveland Department of Veterans Affairs Medical Center by Rice et al [60]. These authors reported an increase in the incidence of ceftazidime-resistant *K pneumoniae* strains from 5% in 1992 to 15% in 1993 to 30% in the first 2 months of 1994. This system-wide outbreak involved the acute care facility and a geographically separate chronic care facility. The highest rates of resistance occurred on the units where ceftazidime was administered most frequently. Molecular epidemiologic studies showed that while plasmid content varied, this was primarily a clonal strain dissemination, based on pulsed-field gel electrophoresis analysis of total genomic DNA. A TEM-6 type ESBL was documented using molecular studies. The institution implemented several control measures. Hospital staff were educated about the problem of ESBL-producing *K pneumoniae* and the association with widespread ceftazidime use, use of ceftazidime was discouraged, piperacillin/tazobactam was added to the formulary, and use of this agent instead of the broad-spectrum cephalosporin was encouraged. Educational measures were successful in changing patterns of antibiotic use without the imposition of antibiotic restrictions. Although this antibiotic use maneuver usually is implemented in conjunction with traditional infection control measures such as Contact Precautions, the primary intervention in this study was a shift from ceftazidime to piperacillin/tazobactam use. Infection control measures such as Contact Precautions were not practical to implement because of the extent of the outbreak. As ceftazidime use decreased and piperacillin/tazobactam use increased, the prevalence of ceftazidime-resistant *K pneumoniae* markedly decreased. Follow-up data documented that ceftazidime-resistant *K pneumoniae* ceased to be a problem at the institution, and piperacillin/tazobactam resistance also decreased in *K pneumoniae*, despite the increase in its use.

A similar experience was noted in San Antonio when an increase in multidrug-resistant *K pneumoniae* was noted in two hospitals within two different patient groups [64]. Similar interventions involving physician education rather than antibiotic restriction resulted in a change in antibiotic usage (decreased ceftazidime use, increased piperacillin/tazobactam use) and an associated decrease in multidrug-resistant *K pneumoniae*. Smith [65] from Indiana reported on the use of a multidisciplinary team that included infection control, infectious diseases, pharmacy, and microbiology to decrease antimicrobial resistance. Interventions included decreased third-generation cephalosporin use, decreased imipenem use, increased extended-spectrum penicillin use, and increased infection control measures. This program was associated with decreased rates of piperacillin resistance in gram-negative bacilli as well as decreased rates of vancomycin-resistant enterococci.

A follow-up study by Rahal and colleagues [66] from the New York institution with the large ESBL *K pneumoniae* outbreak reported initially by Meyer et al [38] noted a gradual increase in the prevalence of these organisms, despite restrictions on third-generation cephalosporin use. Rates of cephalosporin resistance among *K pneumoniae* were approaching 20%, and rates of cephamycin resistance were approaching 40%. The hospital implemented a class restriction of all cephalosporins and cephamycins, with a few exceptions, such as the use of ceftriaxone for meningitis or gonococcal infection. Imipenem restriction was continued. Rates of ceftazidime resistance in *K pneumoniae* and rates of imipenem resistance in *Pseudomonas aeruginosa* were measured in the year before and after the intervention. The cephalosporin restriction measure resulted in an 80% decrease in cephalosporin use throughout the hospital, from 5,558 g/mon to 1,106 g/mon. Imipenem use, however, increased 141% despite restriction, from 197 g/mon to 474 g/mon. A 44% reduction in hospital-acquired ceftazidime-resistant *K pneumoniae* isolates was observed. This decrease was most noticeable in the intensive care units. However, there was a disturbing 69% increase in imipenem-resistant *P aeruginosa* isolates.

Selective Digestive Decontamination

Decre et al [67] from France reported on efforts to use selective digestive decontamination (SDD) in addition to isolation precautions for control of an SHV-4 ESBL *K pneumoniae* outbreak in a medical intensive care unit. An SDD regimen of erythromycin (1 g b.i.d.) and polymyxin E (6 million units b.i.d.) was used initially on all patients admitted to the unit (prophylactic SDD) and then only on colonized or infected patients (curative SDD). Although the prevalence of gastrointestinal colonization decreased nonsignificantly in the prophylactic SDD group, the prevalence of infected patients and the number of extraintestinal sites colonized or infected was higher during the time that prophylactic SDD was used compared with the time that curative SDD was used. Thus, although SDD had an effect on intestinal decontamination, it did not prevent acquisition of ESBL *K pneumoniae*, especially at extraintestinal sites, in the intensive care unit. The authors observed that enhanced adherence to isolation precautions was associated with a reduction in colonization and infection.

Modified Contact Precautions

It is important to increase isolation precautions such as Contact Precautions in the acute care setting, particularly in the intensive care unit, but these types of precautions pose a problem in the chronically ill, another group at risk for multidrug-resistant *K pneumoniae*. We evaluated the prevalence of a multidrug-resistant *K pneumoniae* susceptible only to imipenem and amikacin in a Veterans Affairs-affiliated spinal cord injury center [12]. An initial prevalence survey of 14% colonization or infection with the organism was documented. The major risk factor in this group of patients was chronic urinary catheterization. Modified contact precautions that facilitated rehabilitation goals were employed. Physical and occupational therapy appointments were allowed, and the environment was cleaned vigorously. In addition, a patient and family education program regarding the mode of transmission of multidrug-resistant *K pneumoniae* was implemented. A follow-up prevalence survey 1 year later documented a stable rate at 15% and identified only previously known cases. Thus, modified contact precautions in this chronic care setting prevented dissemination of these organisms in the unit.

Conclusion

The emergence of ESBL-producing *K pneumoniae* and other ESBL-producing *Enterobacteriaceae* is a therapeutic dilemma due to the multiple drug resistance to beta-lactams and other agents, including fluoroquinolones and gentamicin. At this time, imipenem appears to be the drug of choice for serious infections caused by these isolates, based on accumulating clinical experience. Because therapeutic choices are limited, control and prevention measures are especially important. These include traditional infection control measures, such as Contact Precautions, and antibiotic use measures, such as control of widespread use of ceftazidime.

References

1. Shah PW, Stille W. *Escherichia coli* and *Klebsiella pneumoniae* strains more susceptible to cefoxitin than to third generation cephalosporins [letter]. *J Antimicrob Chemother.* 1983;11:597-598.
2. Jarlier V, Nicolas MH, Fournier G, Philippon A. Extended broad-spectrum beta-lactamases confering transferable resistance to newer beta-lactam agents in *Enterobacteriaceae*: hospital prevalence and susceptibility pattern. *Rev Infect Dis.* 1988;10:867-878.
3. Jacoby GA, Medeiros AA, O'Brien TF, Pinto ME, Jiang H. Broad-spectrum, transmissible beta-lactamases. *N Engl J Med.* 1988;319:723-724.
4. Quinn JP, Miyashiro D, Sahm D, Flamm R, Bush K. Novel plasmid-mediated beta-lactamase (TEM-10) conferring selective resistance to ceftazidime and aztreonam in clinical isolates of *Klebsiella pneumoniae. Antimicrob Agents Chemother.* 1989;33:1451-1456.
5. Paterson DL, Ko WC, Mohapatra S, et al. *Klebsiella pneumoniae* bacteremia: impact of extended spectrum beta-lactamase production in a global study of 216 patients. Abstract J210. Presented at the 37th Interscience Congress on Antimicrobial Agents and Chemotherapy, September 28-October 1, 1997, Toronto, Canada.
6. Horii T, Arakawa Y, Ohta M, Ichiyama S, Wacharotayankun R, Kato N. Plasmid-mediated ampC-type beta-lactamase isolated from *Klebsiella pneumoniae* confers resistance to broad-spectrum beta-lactams, including moxalactam. *Antimicrob Agents Chemother.* 1993;37:984-990.
7. Philippon A, Arlet G, Lagrange PH. Origin and impact of plasmid-mediated extended-spectrum beta-lactamases. *Eur J Clin Microbiol Infect Dis.* 1994;13(suppl 1):17-29.
8. Philippon A, Labia R, Jacoby G. Extended-spectrum beta-lactamases. *Antimicrob Agents Chemother.* 1989;33:1131-1136.
9. Jacoby GA, Medeiros AA. More extended-spectrum beta-lactamases. *Antimicrob Agents Chemother.* 1991;35:1697-1704.
10. Medeiros AA. Evolution and dissemination of beta-lactamases accelerated by generations of beta-lactam antibiotics. *Clin Infect Dis.* 1997;24(suppl 1):S19-S45.

11. Ambler RP, Coulson AFW, Frere JM, et al. A standard numbering scheme for the class A beta-lactamases. *Biochem J.* 1991;276:269-270.

12. Przykucki JM, Shoe SL, Patel A, Patterson JE. Prevalence of multi-drug resistant *Klebsiella pneumoniae* in a long term care and spinal cord injury unit. 24th Annual Educational Conference and International Meeting. New Orleans, June 1997.

13. Jacoby GA. Development of resistance in gram-negative pathogens. Extended-spectrum beta-lactamases. In: *Emerging Pathogens in Infectious Disease. A Hospital Practice Special Report.* Minneapolis, Minn: McGraw-Hill; 1999:14-19.

14. Jacoby G, Bush K. Amino acid sequences for TEM, SHV and OXA extended-spectrum and inhibitor resistant beta-lactamases. http://www.lahey.org/studies/webt.htm.

15. Jacoby GA. Extended-spectrum beta-lactamases and other enzymes providing resistance to oxyimino-beta-lactams. *Infect Dis Clin North Am.* 1997;11:875-887.

16. Jacoby GA. The genetics of extended-spectrum beta-lactamases. *Eur J Clin Microbiol Infect Dis.* 1994;13(suppl 1):2.

17. Katsanis GP, Spargo J, Ferraro MJ, Sutton L, Jacoby GA. Detection of *Klebsiella pneumoniae* and *Escherichia coli* strains producing extended-spectrum beta-lactamases. *J Clin Microbiol.* 1994;32:691-696.

18. *National Committee on Clinical Laboratory Standards, M100-S8, 1998.*

19. Sanders CC, Barry AL, Washington JA, et al. Detection of extended-spectrum beta-lactamase-producing members of the family *Enterobacteriaceae* with the VITEK ESBL test. *J Clin Microbiol.* 34:2997-3001.

20. Jacoby GA, Han P. Detection of extended-spectrum beta-lactamases in clinical isolates of *Klebsiella pneumoniae* and *Escherichia coli. J Clin Microbiol.* 1996;34:908-911.

21. Fridkin SK, Gaynes RP. Antimicrobial resistance in intensive care units. *Clin Chest Med.* 1999;20:303-316.

22. http://www.cdc.gov.gov/ncidod/hip/NNIS/AR_Surv1198.pdf

23. Lucet JC, Chevret S, Decre D, et al. Outbreak of multiply resistant *Enterobacteriaceae* in an intensive care unit: epidemiology and risk factors for acquisition. *Clin Infect Dis.* 1996;22:430-436.

24. De Champs C, Rouby D, Guelon D et al. A case-control study of an outbreak of infections caused by *Klebsiella pneumoniae* strains producing CTX-1 (TEM-3) beta-lactamase. *J Hosp Infect.* 1991;18:5-13.

25. Schiappa DA, Hayden MJ, Matushek MG, et al. Ceftazidime-resistant *Klebsiella pneumoniae* and *Escherchia coli* bloodstream infection: a case-control and molecular epidemiologic investigation. *J Infect Dis.* 1996;174:529-536.

26. Pena C, Pujol M, Ardanuy C, et al. Epidemiology and successful control of a large outbreak due to *Klebsiella pneumoniae* producing extended-spectrum beta-lactamases. *Antimicrob Agents Chemother.* 1998;42:53-58.

27. Hibberd PL, Jacoby GA. Multiply drug resistant *Klebsiella pneumoniae* (MDRDP) strains: predictors in acquisition and mortality. Abstract C46. *Abstracts of the 34th Interscience Conference on Antimicrobial Agents and Chemotherapy.* October 4-7, 1994; Orlando, Florida.

28. Piroth L, Aube H, Doise JM, Vincent-Martin M. Spread of extended-spectrum beta-lactamase-producing *Klebsiella pneumoniae*: are beta-lactamase inhibitors of therapeutic value? *Clin Infect Dis.* 1998;27:76-80.

29. Rice LB, Willey SH, Papanicolaou GB, et al. Outbreak of ceftazidime resistance caused by

extended-spectrum beta-lactamases at a Massachusetts chronic-care facility. *Antimicrob Agents Chemother*. 1990;34:2193-2199.

30. Sader HS, Pfaller MA, Jones RN. Prevalence of important pathogens and the antimicrobial activity of parenteral drugs at numerous medical centers in the United States. II. Study of the intra- and interlaboratory dissemination of extended-spectrum beta-lactamase-producing *Enterobacteriaceae*. *Diagn Microbiol Infect Dis*. 1994;20:203-208.

31. Gazouli M, Kaufmann ME, Tzelepi E, Dimopoulou H, Paniara O, Tzouvelekis LS. Study of an outbreak of cefoxitin-resistant *Klebsiella pneumoniae* in general hospital. *J Clin Microbiol*. 1997;35:508-510.

32. Martinez-Martinez L, Hernandes-Alles S, Alberti S, Tomas JM, Benedi VJ, Jacoby GA. In vivo selection of porin-deficient mutants of *Klebsiella pneumoniae* with increased resistance to cefoxitin and expanded-spectrum cephalosporins. *Antimicrob Agents Chemother*. 1996;40:342-348.

33. Martinez-Martinez L, Pascual A, Jacoby GA. Quinolone resistance from a transferable plasmid. *Lancet*. 1998;351:797-799.

34. Jett BD, Ritchie DJ, Reichley R, Bailey TC, Sahm DF. In vitro activities of various beta-lactam antimicrobial agents against clinical isolates of *Escherichia coli* and *Klebsiella* spp. resistant to oxyimino cephalosporins. *Antimicrob Agents Chemother*. 1995;39:1187-1190.

35. Medeiros AA, Creelin J. Comparative susceptibility of clinical isolates producing extended spectrum beta-lactamases to ceftibuten: effect of large inocula. *Pediatr Infect Dis J*. 1997;16:S49-S55.

36. Rice LB, Carias LL, Bonomo RA, Shlaes DM. Molecular genetics of resistance to both ceftazidime and beta-lactam—beta-lactamase inhibitor combinations in *Klebsiella pneumoniae* and in vivo response to beta-lactam therapy. *J Infect Dis*. 1996;173:151-158.

37. Thauvin-Eliopoulos C, Tripodi MF, Moellering RC Jr, Eliopoulos GM. Efficacies of piperacillin-tazobactam and cefepime in rats with experimental intra-abdominal abscesses due to an extended-spectrum beta-lactamase-producing strain of *Klebsiella pneumoniae*. *Antimicrob Agents Chemother*. 1997;41:1053-1057.

38. Meyer KS, Urban C, Eagan JA, Berger BJ, Rahal JJ. Nosocomial outbreak of *Klebsiella* infection resistant to late-generation cephalosporins. *Ann Intern Med*. 1993;119:353-358.

39. Naumovski L, Quinn JP, Miyashiro D, et al. Outbreak of ceftazidime resistance due to a novel extended-spectrum beta-lactamase in isolates from cancer patients. *Antimicrob Agents Chemother*. 1992;36:1991-1996.

40. Karas JA, Pillay DG, Muckart D, Sturm AW. Treatment failure due to extended spectrum beta-lactamase. *J Antimicrob Chemother*. 1996;37:203-204.

41. Pornull KJ, Rodrigo G, Dornbusch K. Production of a plasmid-mediated AmpC-like beta-lactamase by a *Klebsiella pneumoniae* septicaemia isolate. *J Antimicrob Chemother*. 1994;34:943-954.

42. Bradford PA, Urban C, Mariano N, Projan SJ, Rahal JJ, Bush K. Imipenem resistance in *Klebsiella pneumoniae* is associated with the combination of ACT-1, a plasmid-mediated AmpC beta-lactamase, and the loss of an outer membrane protein. *Antimicrob Agents Chemother*. 1997;41:563-569.

43. Pangon B, Bizet C, Bure A, et al. In vivo selection of a cephamycin-resistant, porin-deficient mutant of *Klebsiella pneumoniae* producing a TEM-3 beta-lactamase. *J Infect Dis*. 1989;159:1005-1006.

44. Roussel-Delvallez M, Sirot D, Berrouane Y, et al. Bactericidal effect of beta-lactams and amikacin

alone or in association against *Klebsiella pneumoniae* producing extended spectrum beta-lactamase. *J Antimicrob Chemother.* 1995;36:241-246.

45. Neu HC. Carbapenems. Special properties contributing to their activity. *Am J Med.* 1985;78(suppl 6A):33-40.

46. Senda K, Arakawa Y, Ichiyama S, et al. PCR detection of metallo-beta-lactamase gene (*bla*$_{IMP}$) in gram-negative rods resistant to broad-spectrum beta-lactams. *J Clin Microbiol.* 1996;34:2909-2913.

47. Bingen EH, Desgardins P, Arlet G, et al. Molecular epidemiology of plasmid spread among extended broad-spectrum beta-lactamase-producing *Klebsiella pneumoniae* isolates in a pediatric hospital. *J Clin Microbiol.* 1993;31:179-184.

48. Prodinger WM, Fille M, Bauerfeind A, et al. Molecular epidemiology of *Klebsiella pneumoniae* producing SHV-5 beta-lactamase: parallel outbreaks due to multiple plasmid transfer. *J Clin Microbiol.* 1996;34:564-568.

49. Gori A, Espinasse F, Deplano A, Nonhoff C, Nicolas MH, Struelens MJ. Comparison of pulsed-field gel electrophoresis and randomly amplified DNA polymorphism analysis for typing extended-spectrum-beta-lactamase-producing *Klebsiella pneumoniae*. *J Clin Microbiol.* 1996;334:2448-2453.

50. Marchese A, Arlet G, Schito GC, Langrange PH, Philippon A. Detection of SHV-5 extended-spectrum beta-lactamase in *Klebsiella pneumoniae* strains isolated in Italy. *Eur J Clin Microbiol Infect Dis.* 1996;15:245-248.

51. Branger C, Bruneau B, Lesimple AL, et al. Epidemiological typing of extended-spectrum-beta-lactamase-producing *Klebsiella pneumoniae* isolates responsible for five outbreaks in a university hospital. *J Hosp Infect.* 1997;36:23-36.

52. Rasmussen BA, Bradford PA, Quinn JP, Wiener J, Weinstein RA, Bush K. Genetically diverse ceftazidime-resistant isolates from a single center: biochemical and genetic characterization of TEM-10 beta-lactamases encoded by different nucleotide sequences. *Antimicrob Agents Chemother.* 1993;37:1989-1992.

53. Gouby A, Neuwirth C, Bourg G, et al. Epidemiological study by pulsed-field gel electrophoresis of an outbreak of extended-spectrum beta-lactamase-producing *Klebsiella pneumoniae* in a geriatric hospital. *J Clin Microbiol.* 1994;32:301-305.

54. Bauernfeind A, Rosenthal JE, Eberlein E, Holley M, Schweighart S. Spread of *Klebsiella pneumoniae* producing SHV-5 beta-lactamase among hospitalized patients. *Infection.*1993;21:18-22.

55. Nouvellon M, Pons J-L, Sirot D, Combe J-L, Lemeland J-F. Clonal outbreaks of extended-spectrum beta-lactamase-producing strains of *Klebsiella pneumoniae* demonstrated by antibiotic susceptibility testing, beta-lactamase typing, and multilocus enzyme electrophoresis. *J Clin Microbiol.* 1994;32:2625-2627.

56. French GL, Shannon KP, Simmons N. Hospital outbreak of *Klebsiella pneumoniae* resistant to broad-spectrum cephalosporins and beta-lactam—beta-lactamase inhibitor combinations by hyperproduction of SHV-5 beta-lactamase. *J Clin Microbiol.* 1996;34:358-363.

57. Monnet DL, Biddle JW, Edwards JR, et al. Evidence of interhospital transmission of extended-spectrum beta-lactam-resistant *Klebsiella pneumoniae* in the United States, 1986 to 1993. *Infect Control Hosp Epidemiol.* 1997;18:492-498.

58. Arlet G, Rouveau M, Casin I, Bouvet PJM, Lagrange PH, Philippon A. Molecular epidemiology of *Klebsiella pneumoniae* strains that produce SHV-4 beta-lactamase and which were isolated in 14 French hospitals. *J Clin Microbiol.* 1994;32:2553-2558.

59. Garner JS and the Hospital Infection Control Practices Advisory Committee. Guideline for isolation precautions in hospitals. *Am J Infect Control*. 1996;24:24-52.

60. Rice LB, Eckstein EC, DeVente J, Shlaes DM. Ceftazidime-resistant *Klebsiella pneumoniae* isolates recovered at the Cleveland Department of Veterans Affairs Medical Center. *Clin Infect Dis*. 1996;223:118-124.

61. Urban C, Meyer KS, Mariano N, et al. Identification of TEM-26 beta-lactamase responsible for a major outbreak of ceftazidime-resistant *Klebsiella pneumoniae*. *Antimicrob Agents Chemother*. 1994;28:392.

62. Bradford PA, Cherubin CE, Idemyor V, Rasmussen BA, Bush K. Multiply resistant *Klebsiella pneumoniae* strains from two Chicago hospitals: identification of the extended-spectrum TEM-12 and TEM-10 ceftazidime-hydrolyzing beta-lactamases in a single isolate. *Antimicrob Agents Chemother*. 1994;38:761-766.

63. Brun-Buisson C, Legrand P, Philippon A, Montravers F, Ansquet M, Duval J. Transferable enzymatic resistance to third-generation cephalosporins during nosocomial outbreak of multiresistant *Klebsiella pneumoniae*. *Lancet*. 1987;2:302-306.

64. Patterson JE, Hardin TC, Kelly C, Garcia RC, Jorgensen JH. Association of antibiotic utilization measures and control of multiple drug resistance in extended-spectrum beta-lactamase-producing (ESBL) *Klebsiella pneumoniae*. Abstract 219 *Program and Abstracts of the Infectious Disease Society Annual Meeting*. Denver, Colo:1998.

65. Smith D. Effect of a multidisciplinary team on antimicrobial resistance. *Chest*. In press.

66. Rahal JJ, Urban C, Horn D. Class restriction of cephalosporin use to control total cephalosporin resistance in nosocomial *Klebsiella*. *JAMA*. 1998;280:1233-1237.

67. Decre D, Gachot B, Lucet JC, Arlet G, Bergogne-Berezin E, Regnier B. Clinical and bacteriologic epidemiology of extended-spectrum beta-lactamase-producing strains of *Klebsiella pneumoniae* in a medical intensive care unit. *Clin Infect Dis*. 1998;27:834-844.

Jan E. Patterson, MD, Departments of Medicine (Infectious Diseases) and Pathology, University of Texas Health Science Center at San Antonio, San Antonio, Texas, USA.

IV. *Clostridium difficile* Infection

Donald E. Fry, MD

Clostridium difficile is an anaerobic, gram-positive bacterium that first was identified and characterized in 1935 [1]. Like other *Clostridium* sp, it is a spore-forming microorganism. *C difficile* was accorded little interest until 1978 when several reports identified its association with pseudomembranous enterocolitis [2-6]. Infection with *C difficile* now has become the most common cause of infectious, hospital-acquired diarrhea [7], and the overall frequency of this noso-comial infection appears to be increasing. It is essential that clinicians who care for seriously ill hospitalized patients be sensitive to the clinical presentation, diagnosis, and management of this morbid and occasionally fatal infectious pro-cess.

Epidemiology

C difficile enterocolitis is a disease that occurs primarily in hospitalized pa-tients, particularly among those older than 60 years of age. Current estimates of three million cases per year are interpreted to indicate that *C difficile* is a major nosocomial pathogen in the United States [8]. Only about 20,000 cases per year occur among outpatients [9]. There is a general perception that the total number of *C difficile* infections is increasing, but infection events tend to occur in clus-ters or as acute outbreaks, which makes monitoring of frequency rates within a single or groups of institutions very difficult [10].

Clinical pseudomembranous enterocolitis and antibiotic-associated diarrhea secondary to *C difficile* are most common in the older population. Of interest, healthy neonates and infants may have very high rates of asymptomatic stool colonization ($\geq$50 %) but very low rates of clinical disease [11]. Rates of asymp-tomatic colonization of children diminish rapidly beyond 1 year of age [12]. Up to 3% of asymptomatic adults can be found to have colonization of the stool with *C difficile* [8], although one study from Japan documented a 15% colonization rate [13]. Hospitalized adult patients have rates of colonization of 20% or more [14], and virtually 100% of adult patients with pseudomembanous enterocolitis will have positive stool cultures [6].

The clinically occult nature of asymptomatic stool carriage of *C difficile* is of considerable interest. For many patients, particularly adults, the cultured *C difficile* is not a toxin-producing species, and the absence of clinical infection is attributed to the nonvirulent nature of many cultured strains [15]. However, the recovery of toxin-producing strains from asymptomatic carriers underscores the role of the susceptible host for this infection. Clearly, the presence of the *C difficile* spore in the stool is not necessarily associated with clinical disease; certain host factors promote the transition to the vegetative form of the organism.

For clinical infection with *C difficile* to occur, the patient must have colonic colonization with the organism. As noted previously, a small percentage of patients have such colonization at the time of admission to the hospital, likely due to its ubiquitous presence in soil, water, and other sources. Most patients become colonized after hospitalization due to the presence of spores within the inpatient environment. Spores are shed from both asymptomatic carriers and those who have active disease. The resilience of clostridial spores to common disinfectants makes eradication from the hospital environment very difficult. Hospital personnel are found to have *C difficile* on their hands after they have cared for patients who have clinical infection [14]. Nosocomial transmission to uncolonized patients by breaches in infection control practices is likely to contribute to the development of new cases [16]. Hand washing and liberal use of gloves in all direct patient contacts, especially within the intensive care unit, is necessary to minimize transmission rates.

Natural History and Pathogenesis

Colonization Resistance

Even when the naïve host ingests and becomes colonized with pathogenic *C difficile*, clinical infection may not occur because of the natural host defense mechanism commonly known as colonization resistance. Colonization resistance simply means that the normal qualitative and quantitative components of the human colon prevent the occurrence of clinical infection when the normal colonic ecosystem is challenged with *C difficile* as a new resident [17,18]. While the complete mechanism of colonization resistance is not understood, resident bacteria may produce metabolic products that suppress the growth of pathogenic bacteria or may be more efficient in competing for critical nutrients in the normal environment of the colonic lumen. Enteropathic pathogens need to bind to specific sites on the luminal epithelium cells to create clinical infection, and colonization resistance may result from the large numbers of normal bacteria competitively occupying these potential binding sites. Only when the normal colonization of the colon is disrupted does the pathogen have the opportunity to create clinical infection.

Bacterial Adhesion to Mucosal Cells

Although the specific pathogenesis of *C difficile* enterocolitis has not yet been characterized fully, a reasonable theoretical construct has been hypothesized. Spores of *C difficile* are ingested into the upper digestive tract and survive the hostile acidic gastric environment. If normal colonic colonization has been altered (eg, by systemic antibiotic therapy), the spore can undergo vegetative transformation in the distal small intestine. The *C difficile* bacillus adheres to the gut mucosal cells, which allows proliferation of the organism and production of specific cytotoxins and other virulence factors. Bacteria that fail to adhere to the gut mucosal cells pass harmlessly through the intestinal tract.

Multiple nonspecific defense mechanisms can retard *C difficile* from binding to the mucosal cell surface. Normally produced mucins within the gut retard adherence of pathogenic bacteria. Immunoglobulin A (IgA) antibody can bind to the surface of potential pathogens and prevent adherence [19]. Competing microbial colonists may occupy receptor sites for pathogenic adherence of *C difficile* to the mucosal cells. This competitive inhibition is likely due to native anaerobic colonization and may represent important roles for *Lactobacillus* sp, *Bacteroides* sp, and other normal gut colonists as part of the natural gut barrier [20]. Natural fermentation products of gut anaerobes may prove noxious to potential enteric pathogens [21]. Finally, normal intestinal motility and peristalsis in conjunction with the other host mechanisms can reduce the period of time available for the intraluminal pathogen to adhere to the mucosal cell. Disruption of the normal gut microflora, reduction or elimination of enteral feeding, immunocompromise from severe illness, and sustained ileus are common clinical events that all can contribute to potential enterocolitis with *C difficile*.

C difficile adheres to the enterocyte or colonocyte via specific surface adhesion mechanisms on the bacterial cells. Fimbriae [22] and flagella [23] on the surface of the bacterial cell are potential sources of adhesion, and specific surface proteins on *C difficile* appear to facilitate adhesion [24,25]. The positive charge of the hydrophobic cell surface of *C difficile* may mediate physiochemical adherence to negatively charged gut endothelial cells [26], particularly if competing anaerobic species of the normally colonized host have been altered by antecedent antimicrobial chemotherapy.

Toxin Production

If *C difficile* adhers and proliferates within the distal ileum and colon, toxin production by the pathogen initiates the enterocolitis process. Both a toxin A [27] and a toxin B [28] from *C difficile* have been identified. Toxin A is an enterotoxin and toxin B is a cytotoxin. Both appear to have synergistic effects upon the destruction of gut mucosal cells [29]. Lack of production of these two toxins is seen in nonpathogenic strains of *C difficile* [30].

Injury appears to follow adherence of these toxins to specific receptors on the surface of the host's mucosal cells, and they then are transported into the cytoplasm [31,32]. The absence of toxin receptors on the surface of the immature enterocyte may explain why the neonate who is colonized with toxin-positive bacterial strains does not develop clinical disease [33]. Binding of the enterotoxin to the specific receptor disrupts the normal regulation and control of the cytoskeleton of the cell. "Cell rounding" is seen as evidence of this toxic effect, and cell lysis is the final consequence.

In addition to toxins A and B, *C difficile* has other potential virulence factors that may contribute to clinical disease. Additional toxins of uncertain significance have been identified [34], and hyaluronidase [35] and collagenase [36] are produced by virulent strains. These strains also have a polysaccharide capsule that retards phagocytosis by host neutrophils [37]. Indeed, much of the tissue injury to the distal gut mucosal cells probably is mediated by the severe inflammatory response generated by the host in response to proliferation of the pathogen and its toxins.

Clinical Response

Once infection of the mucosal surface of the distal intestinal tract is established, the combined effects of toxins A and B in concert with the other contributing virulence factors initiates the inflammatory response of the colonic mucosa. The early response is erythema of the mucosa, which is not different in appearance from other nonspecific colitis syndromes. At this point, the patient experiences the first symptoms of diarrhea and crampy abdominal pain. Progression of the disease results in patchy areas of full-thickness mucosal cell death, the appearance of the pseudomembranes that represent areas of fibrinopurulent exudate, and the development of more profound symptoms. Without treatment, the pseudomembranous process proceeds to involve virtually the entire length of the colon, with extensive areas of pseudomembrane formation. Transmural inflammation of the colonic wall leads to dysfunctional colonic peristalsis and the potential development of clinical toxic megacolon. At this point, the patient may have the clinical appearance of severe abdominal pain and systemic toxicity, but diarrhea may cease. Transmural necrosis with or without frank perforation may occur. On occasion, the progression of the colitis can be fulminant, with areas of extensive mucosal necrosis and rapid evolution of a toxic megacolon picture.

Morbidity and Mortality

Although the overall mortality rate from *C difficile* enterocolitis is very low, deaths do occur, usually as a consequence of failure to appreciate symptoms of enterocolitis, with an attendant delay in diagnosis and treatment. In severe cases, continued medical management in the presence of toxic megacolon results in failure to achieve surgical decompression or resection of the severely diseased segments of the colon. Perforation, peritonitis, sepsis, and possibly death can result.

Several studies have addressed the significant costs and patient morbidity that attend toxic megacolon [38-42]. Length of hospitalization for the patient who has *C difficile* enterocolitis is protracted, and selected patients even will suffer clinical relapses that require protracted treatment. A few may require major surgical procedures to address toxic megacolon and even colonic perforations. Early appreciation of the patient at risk and early diagnosis and treatment will minimize both overall costs and patient morbidity.

Risk Factors for Infection

Antibiotic Administration

Antibiotic administration in the period of time leading up to the emergence of *C difficile* infection has been documented in more than 90% of cases. The use of systemic antibiotics is believed to disrupt normal colonization resistance, particularly that provided by normal anaerobic colonization of the gut [43]. Because *Lactobacillus* sp and other gut anaerobes are so exquisitely sensitive to a host of different antibiotics, virtually all antimicrobials have been associated with the development of *C difficile* enterocolitis. Ampicillin, amoxicillin, clindamycin, and cephalosporins are linked most commonly with the development of this infection. Both metronidazole and vancomycin share the dubious distinction of being associated with causing *C difficile* infection, but also being recommended as the preferred choices in treatment of the disease. Sulfonamides, aminoglycosides, ureidopenicillins, and the carbapenems are associated infrequently with *C difficile* infection.

One crossover study examined the impact of specific antibiotic use on the incidence of *C difficile* in two elderly patient tertiary care wards on which there had been outbreaks of *C difficile* colonization and diarrhea [44]. In this prospective, ward-based study, the third-generation cephalosporin cefotaxime was administered empirically in one ward and piperacillin/tazobactam was administered empirically in the matched ward. At the 10-month crossover point, the opposite antibiotic was used for empiric therapy on each ward. There was a highly significant increase in the incidence of *C difficile* colonization (26/34 versus 3/14, *P*=0.001) and diarrhea (18/34 versus 1/14, *P*=0.006) among patients treated with cefotaxime compared with those receiving piperacillin/tazobactam.

Antifungal Chemotherapy

Antifungal chemotherapy with amphotericin B and fluconazole has been associated with *C difficile* infection. However, fungal infections are caused most commonly in hospitalized patients by *Candida albicans,* a microorganism that is associated with antecedent systemic antibiotic therapy and sustained critical illness among patients in the intensive care unit. Most antifungal chemotherapy has little direct impact upon bacterial gut colonization. Thus, the direct effects of amphotericin B or fluconazole upon the incidence of *C difficile* infection in the absence of prior antibacterial antibiotic therapy or severe illness is unclear.

Antiviral Chemotherapy

Antiviral chemotherapy also is associated with *C difficile* infection. As with patients receiving antifungal chemotherapy, those who are being treated with antiviral therapy usually have severe immunosuppression, severe associated illnesses, and commonly have received either antecedent or concurrent antibiotic treatment.

Antineoplastic Chemotherapy

Chemotherapeutic agents for the treatment of cancer have been implicated with *C difficile* infection. Because the patient undergoing aggressive treatment for cancer may be receiving concurrent or recent systemic antibiotic therapy, it has been difficult to establish a clear association. *C difficile* infections have been well documented when no antibiotics were being given to patients receiving anticancer chemotherapy. Most of these patients have been hospitalized for a period of time, so colonization from the hospital environment with *C difficile* and other hospital-acquired organisms is likely. Further, changes in dietary habits, immunosuppression, antacid therapy, and many other variables in the cancer patient may contribute to the disruption of colonization resistance and increased risk of *C difficile* infection. Chemotherapy toxicity affecting the gut mucosa (eg, 5-fluorouracil) may enhance the patient's susceptibility to infection. Radiation therapy without antineoplastic chemotherapy or antibiotics also has been associated with *C difficile* infection.

Elderly Patients/Underlying Disease

Age appears to be a specific risk factor for *C difficile* enterocolitis. One report noted that 80% of positive studies for the enterotoxin of *C difficile* occurred in patients older than age 65 years [45]. Colonization resistance may diminish with the aging process such that lesser antibiotic exposures result in a microenvironment in the colon conducive to enterocolitis. High rates of colonization in patients from extended care facilities and rehabilitation institutions, the disproportionate number of elderly people who have severe illnesses in the intensive care unit, more frequent extended courses of antibiotics, and more common underlying illnesses and immunosuppression offer more opportunities for colonization with *C difficile* among the elderly. The apparent increase of *C difficile* infection in the elderly may be viewed more appropriately as a consequence of underlying disease and higher rates of colonization than as an independent predilection for this infection based solely on age. Underlying illness that compromises host defenses should be viewed in the patient receiving antibiotics as a clinical situation that favors *C difficile* infection regardless of the patient's age.

Ulcerative colitis, perhaps regional enteritis, and chemotherapeutic-induced enterocolitis appear to be associated with increased rates of *C difficile* infection. Cancer patients in general, renal dialysis patients, and patients who have other clinical evidence of protein-calorie malnutrition appear unusually susceptible to this infection. Increased duration of hospital stay similarly increases the risk of *C difficile* colonization.

Postoperative Patients

Increased rates of *C difficile* infection have been identified among postoperative patients, particularly following gastrointestinal operations. These patients may be at increased risk because the commonly used nasogastric tube may be an unusually efficient portal to the alimentary tract for spores. Gastrointestinal surgical patients typically have preoperative bowel preparation, receive oral preoperative antibiotics that are poorly absorbed, experience impaired motility secondary to ileus, receive systemic perioperative antibiotic prophylaxis, and have variable lengths of no oral caloric intake during the postoperative period.

The continued imprudent use of prolonged postoperative systemic antibiotics for presumed preventive purposes, particularly among the elderly and patients who have nasogastric tubes (or other enteric tubes) appears to be a recipe for preventable infections with *C difficile*.

Poor Infection Control Practices

The colonization of patients with the spore of *C difficile* probably is aided by breaches of standard practices of infection control. Failure to wash hands routinely between patient contacts means that infections due to *C difficile*, methicillin-resistant *Staphylococcus aureus*, and vancomycin-resistant *Enterococcus* sp likely will continue to be major problems in the intensive care unit. Transmission of the spores through contaminated equipment and even casual transmission from hand contact with contaminated equipment is understandable because of the persistence of the spore. Greater use of disposable gloves when handling bed linen and all physical contacts with contaminated patients in the intensive care unit is essential. There is little evidence that the spore of *C difficile* is transmitted by airborne routes in sufficient numbers to cause clinical infection. Contaminated hands, surfaces, and equipment may account for colonization of many patients.

Diagnosis

Signs and Symptoms

Classic signs and symptoms make the diagnosis of *C difficile* infection readily apparent in many patients. The disease may present in any of five different patterns: 1) asymptomatic carriage, 2) colitis syndrome without pseudomembranes, 3) colitis with pseudomembranes, 4) toxic megacolon, and 5) fulminant colitis. The severity of the disease usually depends on the duration of infection, but it also may reflect a large inoculum of colonization in an unusually susceptible host who has numerous risk factors.

Asymptomatic carriage of this bacterium is recognized among hospitalized adult patients, but its clinical significance in the absence of symptoms is unclear [46]. Patients who develop *C difficile* infection following discharge from the hospital likely were asymptomatically colonized during their hospitalization. The exact percentage of patients who are colonized with *C difficile* remains difficult to define because of the number of risk factors present in any given patient, the high variability of infection in different institutions, and the need to culture the organism rather than to detect toxin to establish the state of asymptomatic carriage. Identification of those who are asymptomatic carriers may have some epidemiologic value in identifying patterns of spread and risk for infection or possibly the risk for patients who may be continued on antibiotics after discharge from the hospital. Obtaining stool cultures from high-risk patients is not recommended at this time.

Diarrhea is the cardinal symptom that signals the diagnosis of *C difficile* enterocolitis. It should be emphasized that hospitalized patients have several reasons to develop a diarrhea syndrome, and only 30% of hospital-associated diarrhea syndromes will be positive for *C difficile* infection, even in an environment that has a high incidence of this infection (Table IV-1) [47]. Diarrhea has been defined as six watery stools over 36 hours, three unformed stools over 24 hours for 2 days, or eight unformed stools over 48 hours [48-50]. Obviously, objective criteria defining diarrhea are "soft," but multiple episodes of presumed diarrhea or unformed stools over a 24-hour period of time should stimulate further diagnostic assessment. Bloody diarrhea is uncommon with *C difficile* enterocolitis, and gross blood that is identified in the bowel movement favors other diagnostic possibilities. In addition to diarrhea, other clinical symptoms suggestive of *C difficile* enterocolitis include crampy abdominal pain, anorexia, and perhaps mild fever and leukocytosis. In patients with pseudomembranes and those with unusually severe cases of enterocolitis, severe consequences of diarrhea include dehydration, hypoalbuminemia, and other electrolyte abnormalities.

Proctosigmoidoscopy commonly is undertaken at the onset of the diarrhea syndrome. The presence of pseudomembranes over the colonic surface is not a requirement for the diagnosis of enterocolitis [51], but it does confirm the diagnosis. Pseudomembrane formation is uncommon with other causes of hospital-associated diarrhea. The pseudomembranous exudate is visual testimony to the severity of the infection or to the duration of the enterocolitis. Promptly recognized and diagnosed enterocolitis will not have pseudomembranous changes and likely will respond more promptly to treatment. In a small percentage of patients, the pseudomembranous changes may be in the more proximal segments of the colon and outside the length of the proctosigmoidoscope [52].

Laboratory Evaluation

The diagnosis of *C difficile* enterocolitis is best made by detection of the toxin within a specimen of diarrheal stool. A host of different enzyme-linked immunosorbent assays (ELISAs) are used that employ either monoclonal or polyclonal antibodies [53,54]. Most commonly the antibodies are directed toward the detection of toxin A. Numerous commercial kits are available for the detection of these toxins and have reported sensitivities for detection of toxins of

Table IV-1. Potential Causes for Diarrhea in a Patient in the Intensive Care Unit

- Medications
  - Angiotensin-converting enzyme inhibitors
  - Antineoplastic agents
  - Beta-blockers
  - Digoxin
  - Diuretics
  - Histamine blockers
  - Magnesium antacids
  - Misoprostol
  - Procainamide
  - Quinidine
  - Sorbitol
  - Theophylline
- Infections
  - *Clostridium difficile*
  - *Campylobacter* sp
  - *Escherichia coli*
  - *Salmonella* sp
  - *Shigella* sp
  - *Yersinia* sp
- Enteral feeding
- Fecal impaction
- Ischemic colitis
- Internal intestinal fistula
- Pancreatic insufficiency

65% to 95% and specificity for *C difficile* toxins of 75% to 100% [55]. ELISA studies for toxin should be performed only on diarrheal stools; false-positive findings can occur in up to 10% of formed stool specimens [56]. The fresh specimen should be stored at 4°C if the assay is not performed immediately [57]. Specimens can be stored for 24 hours without affecting the accuracy of the study. The impression in reviewing all of the diagnostic kits is that those designed to detect both toxins A and B have greater clinical accuracy than those designed to detect toxin A alone [58]. Examination of three separately obtained specimens appears to improve overall accuracy in detecting the toxin by about 10% [59], although routine use of three separate specimens should be discouraged for most patients.

Because both false-positive and false-negative findings are obtained with detection of toxin in the stool, other diagnostic methods have been evaluated. The latex agglutination method has been used to detect glutamate dehydrogenase in stool [60]. It has less specificity and sensitivity than does ELISA for establishing the diagnosis, and colonization of the colon with nontoxigenic species of *C difficile* will result in false-positive findings. For these reasons, this study is not used commonly, even though it is less expensive and easily performed.

Direct recovery of the *C difficile* organism by culture isolation has been common practice for epidemiologic study of these infections. However, culturing of anaerobic species has proven difficult for many laboratories and because sensitivities play no practical role in the selection of antibiotic therapy, only toxin detection is considered a clinically necessary diagnostic study. The common culture method uses an egg yolk agar that contains cycloserine, cefoxitin, and fructose [61]. The plated culture medium is incubated under anaerobic conditions. *C difficile* is consistently resistant to cefoxitin; other colonic anaerobes are suppressed by its use in the culture medium. Numerous variations have been employed in the culture medium to improve recovery of *C difficile* from the clinical specimen [62,63]. Some believe that recovery of the pathogen by culture identification is the most accurate method for establishing the diagnosis [64,65], but the complexity of the culturing process has limited its use in most clinical laboratories. Further, recovery of *C difficile* in the stool does not identify whether the isolate is a toxin-producing species.

The cytotoxicity assay assesses toxic effects of stool filtrates [54,66]. Different cell culture lines are used, and the stool filtrate is incubated overnight in tissue culture to document the "rounding" cell response from cytotoxic effects. Careful dilution of the stool specimen for tissue culture is critical for performing this assay because excessive or inadequate dilution can give false-positive or false-negative results. When performed correctly, this study may be the most accurate for toxin detection because it is a biologic assay of actual cytotoxic effect [64]. However, it is expensive and technically demanding and is not currently performed outside of research settings.

Direct identification of the gene from either toxin A or B in the stool specimen holds new promise for diagnosing *C difficile* enterocolitis [67-69]. The polymerase chain reaction is used to amplify the toxin-producing genes. The cost, technical complexity, and overall sensitivity of this technique require significant improvement before it can become a practical study for general clinical use.

Other diagnostic methods have been used in the past, but are now abandoned. Gram stains and fecal leukocyte counts performed on the diarrheal specimen lack specificity [70]. Detection of blood in the stool is not useful because most patients with *C difficile* enterocolitis have no occult blood in the specimen [47]. Electrophoretic [71] and chromatographic [72] methods to detect toxin or characteristic markers (eg, fatty acids) to serve as diagnostic surrogates for *C difficile* have no clinical value.

The direct detection of toxin in the stool specimen by ELISA remains the most commonly accepted study. When the variables of specificity, sensitivity, cost, rapidity of performance, and technical ease of performance are considered, direct toxin detection appears to be the most practical diagnostic method [73].

Radiographic Evaluation

Radiographic studies offer little diagnostic value for routine *C difficile* enterocolitis; abdominal roentgenograms will provide only nonspecific findings. However, radiographic studies assume greater value when enterocolitis evolves into toxic megacolon. Undiagnosed and untreated enterocolitis can evolve into transmural extension of the inflammatory process with attendant failure of normal colonic motility. The abdomen distends progressively, and the frequency and severity of diarrhea decreases. Abdominal tenderness with rebound develops, and patients may have a systemic clinical pattern of sepsis. Abdominal roentgenograms demonstrate generalized colonic and specifically cecal dilatation not unlike that seen in Ogilvie's syndrome or in patients who have advanced ulcerative colitis. Small bowel air-fluid levels that are analogous to that seen with mechanical small bowel obstruction are evident. Abdominal computed tomography (CT), which is essentially of no value for the typical case of *C difficile* enterocolitis, will demonstrate thickening of the colonic wall, mucosal "thumbprinting," and even an "accordion" appearance if gastrointestinal contrast is used with the study [74,75]. Ascites may or may not be present.

Occasionally, patients may have a fulminant enterocolitis syndrome from *C difficile* infection that is associated with only a transient period of diarrhea or no diarrhea [76]. The fulminant infection presents with obstipation, abdominal distention, and abdominal pain and tenderness. These patients will demonstrate colonic distention and CT findings as noted with toxic megacolon. Because many of these patients are postoperative, there may be confusion about whether they have a postoperative ileus. Older patients may be viewed as having Ogilvie's syndrome. The diagnosis can be difficult to establish because few diarrheal specimens are available for toxin assay. Furthermore, proctosigmoidoscopy or colonoscopy must be approached with caution to avoid perforation. Pseudomembranes can be visualized and colonic contents sampled for toxin assays via endoscopy [77]. It is most important to appreciate that the elderly surgical patient receiving systemic antibiotic therapy is at risk for *C difficile* entero-colitis even when the number of unformed stools is small or when the patient has acute onset of abdominal distention, pain, or tenderness without diarrhea. A high index of suspicion is necessary and may even require empirical therapy in selected patients because of the problems in obtaining either visual or toxin docu-mentation.

Therapy

Treatment of *C difficile* enterocolitis focuses on three basic strategies. First, the antibiotic therapy that has mediated the change in the patient's colonic mi-croflora should be discontinued or it should be changed to drugs that have less of an association with enterocolitis. As noted earlier, *C difficile* clinical isolates are resistant to cephalosporins, and these antibiotics have a strong association with the development of enterocolitis. Similarly, clindamycin, ampicillin, and amoxicillin therapy should be discontinued or changed to an alternative without strong associations with enterocolitis. Continuation of antibiotics that foster *C difficile* enterocolitis may delay clinical resolution of the disease when appro-priate therapy is initiated and may contribute to recidivism of the infection after an initial response to specific antimicrobial therapy.

Second, antiperistaltic medications should be avoided [78]. Diarrhea is the response of the infected host to expel pathogens responsible for enterocolitis. Use of antiperistaltic medications results in retention of the pathogen, probably worsens enterocolitis-associated necrosis of the colonic mucosa, and increases the risk of colonic dysmotility and toxic megacolon [79]. Clinical resolution of the acute enterocolitis syndrome is identified best as cessation of the diarrheal syndrome following the initiation of appropriate antimicrobial therapy, and ag-gressive use of antiperistaltic agents leave uncertainty about the effectiveness of therapy. Because of the loss of fluid and electrolytes with the diarrhea and extra-cellular losses of volume into the inflamed soft tissues of the colon, extracellular water and electrolyte replacement must be administered by the intravenous route until the diarrhea has ceased and effective oral intake has resumed.

Third, specific antibiotic therapy to treat the offending *C difficile* pathogen should be initiated. Either vancomycin or metronidazole is recommended. Com-parative trials of these antimicrobials at appropriate doses have demonstrated comparable efficacy. However, specific features of these drugs affect the choice [80,81]. One principle of therapy has been to use an oral antimicrobial to treat enterocolitis. Little of orally administered vancomycin is absorbed, and it re-sults in very high concentrations within the colonic lumen. Proximal absorption of metronidazole is efficient. Its clinical effectiveness is related to its elimination in active form within the bile and its systemic delivery to the active infection within the colonic mucosa. Therapeutic concentrations are achieved within the colonic lumen even though little of the drug remains unabsorbed after oral administration.

A third potential choice in the treatment of *C difficile* enterocolitis is oral teicoplanin or bacitracin. Teicoplanin has considerable in vitro activity against *C difficile*, but it has not been shown to be clinically superior to vancomycin [81]. Bacitracin is active against *C difficile*, although initial response rates are lower, and recurrence rates are higher than with either metronidazole or vancomycin [82].

Severe infections and cases with elements of gut dysmotility and toxic megacolon may require intravenous therapy [83]. Intravenous administration of vancomycin is thought to provide poorer drug concentrations at the site of infection than oral treatment. However, *C difficile* is exquisitely sensitive to vancomycin at very low concentrations. Nevertheless, when intravenous therapy is required, most clinicians prefer metronidazole because it appears that higher drug concentrations can be achieved [84] and excretion of the drug via the bile may afford better intraluminal concentrations [85].

The emergence of vancomycin-resistant *Enterococcus* sp as nosocomial pathogens in the intensive care unit have raised concerns about the use of this drug. Increased use of systemic vancomycin for the treatment of infections caused by methicillin-resistant staphylococci and for empirical therapy in the intensive care unit has been directly associated with the emergence of the vancomycin-resistant enterococci. Oral vancomycin has similarly been implicated [86]. Thus, many infection control officers are recommending the use of vancomycin only when there are no other treatment alternatives (eg, methicillin-resistant staphylococci). Metronidazole is the preferred treatment of choice for *C difficile* enterocolitis in institutions where the emergence of vancomycin-resistant enterococci is an established problem.

A final consideration in the choice of treatment is cost. Metronidazole is very inexpensive. Vancomycin is extremely expensive. Oral vancomycin preparations are especially expensive because there are essentially no indications for their use other than enterocolitis. A 10-day oral course of vancomycin has been estimated to be 100-fold more costly than a similar oral course of metronidazole [87].

The dosing and duration of antimicrobial therapy also are interesting considerations in these patients. It is estimated that nearly 25% of patients who have mild enterocolitis will recover following discontinuation of the offending antibiotic without treatment specifically targeted for *C difficile* [80]. Metronidazole is administered at a dose of 250 to 500 mg four times per day for 10 to 14 days [80]. The vancomycin dosage schedule is 125 mg four times per day for 10 to 14 days [82,88]. Recurrence of infection occurs less commonly with courses of treatment that last 10 days or longer [87]. However, infection recurrence due to perceived persistence of *C difficile* colonization occurs in 20% to 30% of patients who receive appropriate treatment [89,90]. Monitoring for the presence of toxin in the colon is not helpful in predicting either successful therapy or recurrence of infection following an apparently successful course of treatment because many patients remain toxin-positive after clinical infection resolves and without identification of posttreatment clinical recurrence.

Recurrent Infection

Recurrent symptoms from toxin-positive diarrhea after apparently successful initial treatment are associated with a history of previous episodes of enterocolitis, continued or interval antibiotic therapy for another infection with drugs that have a strong association with this infection, and with specific strains of *C difficile* [91]. Recurrent infection is not associated with resistance to the antimicrobial therapy used to treat the enterocolitis, but it may be associated with therapy that was too short in duration. Interestingly, many recurrent infections are attributed to a different strain of *C difficile* from that causing the initial infection [92].

Treatment of recurrent infection requires resumption of therapy. Oral metronidazole 250 to 500 mg four times per day is recommended. If the patient does not respond within 48 hours, vancomycin therapy should be implemented [93]. More than 90% of patients experience complete resolution of the enterocolitis without further recurrences [83]. Multiply recurrent infections occur in a small number of patients, and they pose a difficult treatment challenge. Potential but as yet unproven strategies for managing this group of patients are summarized in Table IV-2.

Surgical Indications

Selected patients with severe toxic megacolon or acute fulminant colitis may be refractory to medical management. Invasive infection, necrosis of mucosa, stasis of colonic contents due to dysmotility, and increased intraluminal pressure result in transmural necrosis and even colonic perforation. A critical point is reached in patient management when surgical intervention must be considered.

Table IV-2. Potential Treatment Strategies for Multiply Recurrent *C difficile* Enterocolitis

Treatment	Reference	Comment
Tapered vancomycin dosing	Tedesco et al [94]	Presumes that prolonged antibiotic therapy will allow clearance of colonic colonization
Vancomycin plus rifampin	Buggy et al [95]	Attempts to clear colonization with synergistic effects of combination therapy
Vancomycin followed by cholestyramine	Moncino et al [96] Kreutzer and Milligan [97]	Cholestyramine may bind toxin, but it also may bind vancomycin [98]
Vancomycin followed by *Saccharomyces boulardii*	Surawicz et al [99] McFarland et al [100]	Strategy restores "colonization resistance" with competing organism; digestion of toxin by yeast may be an additional mechanism [101]
Metronidazole or bacitracin followed by *Lactobacillus* sp	Gorbach et al [102] Biller et al [103]	Restores colonization resistance with competing organism
Vancomycin followed by fecal bacterial enema	Tvede et al [104] Schwan et al [105]	Restores colonization with normal fecal flora
Nontoxigenic *C difficile*	Seal et al [106]	Competitive inhibition of pathogenic species for colonocyte binding sites
Enterococcus faecium SF 68	Lewenstein et al [107]	Restores colonization resistance with competing organism
Yogurt	Siitonen et al [108]	Restores colonization resistance with competing organisms
Brewer's yeast	Schellenberg et al [109]	Restores colonization resistance with competing organisms

Table IV-2. Potential Treatment Strategies for Multiply Recurrent *C difficile* Enterocolitis (cont)

Treatment	Reference	Comment
Immune globulin and *Saccharomyces boulardii*	Hassett et al [110]	Eliminates chronic colonization and restores colonization resistance
Anti-*C difficile* bovine immunoglobulin	Kelly et al [111,112]	Passive immunity to eliminate chronic colonization
Intravenous gamma globulin	Leung et al [113]	Passive immunity to eliminate chronic colonization

Failure of colonic distention to respond to medical management, cecal distention greater than 10 cm, a progressive septic picture, and evidence of multiple organ failure in the face of appropriate antimicrobial therapy suggest the need for abdominal exploration. Evidence of bowel perforation and diffuse rebound tenderness also warrant abdominal exploration. Failure to pursue timely surgical intervention when appropriate will result in death from this infection.

The choice of the surgical procedure depends on findings at the time of surgical exploration. If transmural necrosis is identified, all necrotic colon should be resected. Proximal colostomy and a distal Hartmann pouch will be necessary. Left hemicolectomy is usually the minimum procedure required and is appropriate if the proximal line of resection extends to the right transverse colon. It provides optimum perfusion of the colostomy at the site of the middle colic artery. The presence of necrotic mucosa warrants subtotal colectomy. It is important to emphasize that necrotic mucosa has a viable seromuscular coat. Necrotic tissue in the line of resection of the left hemicolectomy is an indication to extend the resection. Excision of all colon that has transmural necrosis or necrotic mucosa in the sigmoid colon usually precludes the ability to bring out a mucus fistula. Overall best results for these patients are achieved with subtotal colectomy with ileostomy [75,114,115].

Prevention

Strategies to prevention *C difficile* enterocolitis focus on reducing patient-to-patient spread of *C difficile* and the hospital reservoir as a source of the spores through disinfection and cleaning policies. Prevention also requires major changes in the clinical practice of using antibiotics.

Transmission of *C difficile* between and among patients in specialty and intensive care units has been documented to be a source of enterocolitis [116]. Hand washing between patient contacts must be emphasized continually. Gloves must be used in handling linen, body fluids, and equipment from patients who have established infection. Although difficult to prove, systematic and comprehensive disinfection of facilities and equipment used in the care of patients known to have enterocolitis should minimize the risks of transfer to new patients [117,118]. Cohorting or isolating patients who have active infection has been difficult to validate as a preventive measure, but it makes clinical sense, particularly in facilities that have a high incidence of these infections [119,120]. Antimicrobial treatment of asymptomatic carriers of *C difficile* proven by toxin assays has been shown to have a favorable impact on new cases when vancomycin was used [121], but it was not effective with metronidazole [122].

Reducing the adverse effects of systemic antibiotics must be an objective for prevention. Reduced use of drugs that are strongly associated with enterocolitis when alternative choices are available is desirable. A shorter duration of antibiotic administration and less use of combination antibiotics will help to prevent enterocolitis [123] and reduce the general stress on antimicrobial resistance profiles within the intensive care unit. Finally, it is important to avoid anaerobic antibiotics in the management of intensive care unit nosocomial infection unless anaerobes can be clearly shown to participate in the infection.

Perhaps the greatest area for reduced antibiotic use that will translate into a reduced incidence of *C difficile* enterocolitis is the use of preventive antibiotics in surgery. The clear evidence of three decades of clinical research documents that preventive antibiotics will reduce infection at the surgical site when present within the tissues at the time of the procedure and the contamination. Prolonged administration of antibiotics in the postoperative period after wound closure has no impact upon the frequency of surgical site infection. Further, prolonged administration of preventive antibiotics after elective surgery is associated with increased case rates of enterocolitis and is a prime area for practice changes that can reduce the frequency of this complication [124]. Institutional stop orders and strong administrative enforcement of compliance with standard practices in this and other areas may become necessary [125].

Future Problems and Directions

The aging of society and the sophistication of supportive care measures means that large numbers of patients with risk factors for *C difficile* enterocolitis will continue to receive care in the intensive care unit. The management of community-acquired and hospital-acquired infection will continue to require systemic antimicrobial therapy. Antibiotic resistance and older, sicker patients means that combination antibiotic therapy will continue to be necessary. All of these factors suggest that *C difficile* enterocolitis will continue to be a problem. If resistance emerges to metronidazole and vancomycin, the management of acute and recurrent enterocolitis will enter a new dimension of complexity.

Fundamental to future strategies for preventing and treating *C difficile* enterocolitis is a better understanding of colonization resistance and the roles of antibiotics, aging, and other variables in changing the colonic milieu. Preserving or restoring the resistance of the colon to enterocolitis must be the direction of new research and new treatment. It is not realistic to think that *C difficile* will be eradicated or that resistance of this organism to current antimicrobial therapy will not develop. Newer therapies, many of which are being explored (Table IV-2), are seeking methods to repopulate the normal gut colonization (eg, through nutrient delivery systems or administering biotherapy with "friendly" bacteria or yeast). Because *C difficile* infection is both initiated and treated by antibiotics, future prevention and treatment strategies likely will focus on administering bacteria or preserving bacterial colonization rather than eradicating the pathogen with yet more antimicrobial therapy.

References

1. Hall JC, O'Toole. Intestinal flora in new-borne infants with a description of a new pathogenic anaerobe, *Bacillus difficiles*. *Am J Dis Child*. 1935;49:390-402.
2. Bartlett JG, Chang TW, Gurwith T, et al. Antibiotic-associated pseudomembranous colitis due to toxin-producing clostridia. *N Engl J Med*. 1978;298:531-534.
3. Bartlett JG, Moon N, Chang TW, et al. Role of *Clostridium difficile* in antibiotic-associated pseudomembranous colitis. *Gastroenterology*. 1978;75:778-782.
4. George RH, Symonds JM, Dimock F, et al. Identification of *Clostridium difficile* as a cause of pseudomembranous colitis. *Br Med J*. 1978;1:695.
5. George WL, Sutter VL, Finegold SM. Toxigenicity and antimicrobial susceptibility of *Clostridium difficile*, a cause of antimicrobial agent-associated colitis. *Curr Microbiol*. 1978;1:55-58.
6. Larson HE, Price AB, Honour P, Borriello SP. *Clostridium difficile* and the aetiology of pseudomembranous colitis. *Lancet*. 1978;1:1063-1066.
7. Ringel AF, Jameson GL, Foster ES. Diarrhea in the intensive care patient. *Crit Care Clin*. 1995;11:465-477.

8. Kelly CP, LaMont JT. *Clostridium difficile* infection. *Annu Rev Med*. 1998;49:375-390.
9. Hirschhorn LR, Trnka Y, Onderdonk A, et al. Epidemiology of community-acquired *Clostridium difficile*-associated diarrhea. *J Infect Dis*. 1994;169:127-133.
10. Biordon DW. *Clostridium difficile*: the epidemiology and prevention of hospital-acquired infection. *Infection*. 1982;10:203-204.
11. Larson HE, Barclay FE, Honour P, Hill ID. Epidemiology of *Clostridium difficile* in infants. *J Infect Dis*. 1982;146:727-733.
12. Viscidi R, Wiley S, Bartlett JG. Isolation rates and toxigenic potential of *Clostridium difficile* isolates from various patient populations. *Gastroenterology*. 1981;81:5-9.
13. Nakamura S, Mikawa M, Takabataki M, et al. Isolation of *Clostridium difficile* from the feces and antibody sera of young and elderly adults. *Microbiol Immunol*. 1981;25:345-351.
14. McFarland LV, Mulligan ME, Kwok RYY, Stamm WE. Nosocomial acquisition of *Clostridium difficile* infection. *N Engl J Med*. 1989;320:204-210.
15. Bartlett JG. *Clostridium difficile*: history of its roles as an enteric pathogen and the current state of knowledge about the organism. *Clin Infect Dis*. 1994;18(suppl 4):S265-S272.
16. Nolan NPM, Kelly CP, Humphreys JFH, et al. An epidemic of pseudomembranous colitis: importance of person-to-person spread. *Gut*. 1987;28:1467-1473.
17. Wilson KH. The microecology of *Clostridium difficile*. *Clin Infect Dis*. 1993;16(suppl 4):S214-S218.
18. Borrielo SP. Pathogenesis of *Clostridium difficile* infection. *J Antimicrob Chemother*. 1998;41(suppl C):13-19.
19. Guerrant RL, Bobak DA. Bacterial and protozoal gastroenteritis. *N Engl J Med*. 1991;325:327-340.
20. Borriello SP. The influence of the normal flora on *Clostridium difficile* colonisation of the gut. *Ann Med*. 1990;22:61-67.
21. Rolfe RD. Role of volatile fatty acids in colonization resistance to *Clostridium difficile*. *Infect Immun*. 1984;45:185-191.
22. Borriello SP, Davies HA, Barclay FE. Detection of fimbrae among strains of *Clostridium difficile*. *FEMS Microbiol Lett*. 1988;49:65-67.
23. Tasteyre A, Barc MC, Dodson P, et al. Isolation of a genetic determinant coding for *Clostridium difficile* flagellin and its relation to different serotypes. *Bioscience Microflora*. 1997;16(suppl):19.
24. Evillard M, Fourel V, Barc MC, et al. Identification and characterization of adhesive factors of *Clostridium difficile* involved in adhesion to human colonic enterocyte-like Caco-2 and mucus-secreting HT29 cells in culture. *Molecular Microbiol*. 1993;7:371-381.
25. Karjalainen T, Barc MC, Collignon A, et al. Cloning of a genetic determinant from *Clostridium difficile* involved in adherence to tissue culture cells and mucus. *Infect Immun*. 1994;62:4347-4355.
26. Krishna MM, Powell NBL, Borriello SP. Cell surface properties of *Clostridium difficile*: haemmagglutination, relative hydrophobicity and charge. *J Med Microbiol*. 1996;44:115-123.
27. Dove CH, Wang SZ, Price SB, et al. Molecular characterization of the *Clostridium difficile* toxin A gene. *Infect Immun*. 1990;58:480-488.
28. Barroso LA, Wang SZ, Phelps CJ, et al. Nucleotide sequence of the *Clostridium difficile* toxin B gene. *Nucleic Acids Res*. 1990;18:4004.
29. Lyerly DM, Saum KE, MacDonald DK, Wilkins TD. Effects of *Clostridium difficile* toxins given intragastrically to animals. *Infect Immun*. 1985;47:349-352.

30. Fekety R, Shah AB. Diagnosis and treatment of *Clostridium difficile* colitis. *JAMA*. 1993;269:71-75.

31. Pothoulakis C, LaMont JT, Eglow R, et al. Characterization of rabbit ileal receptors for *Clostridium difficile* toxin A: evidence for a receptor-coupled G protein. *J Clin Invest*. 1991; 88:119-125.

32. Hecht G, Pothoulakis C, LaMont JT, Madara JL. *Clostridium difficile* toxin A perturbs cytoskeletal structure and tight junction permeability of cultured human intestinal epithelial monolayers. *J Clin Invest*. 1988;82:1516-1524.

33. Eglow R, Pothoulakis C, Itzkowitz S, et al. Diminished *Clostridium difficile* toxin A sensitivity in newborn rabbit ileus is associated with decreased toxin A receptor. *J Clin Invest*. 1992;90:822-829.

34. Borriello SP, Davies HA, Kamiya S, et al. Virulence factors of *Clostridium difficile*. *Rev Infect Dis*. 1990;12(suppl 2):S185-S191.

35. Hafiz S, Oakley CL. *Clostridium difficile*: isolation and characteristics. *J Med Microbiol*. 1976;9:129-136.

36. Seddon SV, Hemingway I, Borriello SP. Hydrolytic enzyme production by *Clostridium difficile* and its relationship to toxin production production and virulence in the hamster model. *J Med Microbiol*. 1990; 31:169-174.

37. Davies HA, Borriello SP. Detection of capsule in strains of *Clostridium difficile* of varying virulence and toxigenicity. *Microb Pathogen*. 1990;9:141-146.

38. Cartmell TDI, Panigrahi H, Worsley MA, et al. Management and control of a large outbreak of diarrhea due to *Clostridium difficile*. *J Hosp Infect*.1994;27:1-15.

39. Macgowan AP, Brown I, Feeney R, et al. *Clostridium difficile* associated diarrhoea and length of hospital stay. *J Hosp Infect*. 1995;31:241-244.

40. Riley TV, Codde JP, Rouse IL. Increased length of stay due to *Clostridium difficile* associated diarrhoea. *Lancet*. 1995;345:455-456.

41. Wilcox MH, Cunniffe JG, Trundle C, Redpath C. Financial burden of hospital-acquired *Clostridium difficile* infection. *J Hosp Infect*. 1996;34:23-30.

42. Kofsky P, Rosen L, Reed J, et al. *Clostridium difficile*: a common and costly colitis. *Dis Colon Rectum*. 1991;34:244-248.

43. Vollaard EJ, Clasener HAL, van Saene HKF, et al. Effect of colonization resistance: an important criterion in selecting antibiotics. *DICP: Anu Pharmacother*. 1990;24:60-66.

44. Settle CD, Wilcox MH, Fawley WN, Corrado OJ, Hawkey PM. Prospective study of the risk of *Clostridium difficile* diarrhoea in elderly patients following treatment with cefotaxime or piperacillin/tazobactam. *Aliment Pharmacol Ther*. 1998;12:1217-1223.

45. Communicable Disease Surveillance Center. *Clostridium difficile* in England and Wales: quarterly report. *Communicable Disease Report Weekly*. 1997;7:412.

46. Johnson S, Clabots CR, Linn FV, et al. Nosocomial *Clostridium difficile* colonisation and disease. *Lancet*. 1990;336:97-100.

47. Gerding DN, Olson MM, Peterson LR, et al. *Clostridium difficile*-associated diarrhea and colitis in adults: a prospective case-controlled epidemiologic study. *Arch Intern Med*. 1986;146:95-100.

48. Shanholtzer CJ, Willard KE, Holter JJ, et al. Comparison of VIDAS *C difficile* toxin A imunoassay (CDA) with *C difficile* culture, cytotoxin, and latex test. *J Clin Microbiol*. 1992;30:1837-1840.

49. McFarland LV, Mulligan M, Kwok RYY, Stamm WE. Nosocomial acquisition of *Clostridium difficile* infection. *N Engl J Med*. 1989;320:204-210.

50. Walker RC, Ruane PJ, Rosenblatt JE, et al. Comparison of culture, cytotoxicity assays, and

enzyme-linked immunosorbent assay for toxin A and toxin B in the diagnosis of *Clostridium difficile*-related enteric disease. *Diag Microbiol Infect Dis.* 1986; 5:61-69.

51. Bergstein JM, Kramer A, Wittman DH, et al. Pseudomembranous colitis: how useful is endoscopy? *Surg Endoscopy.* 1990;4:217-219.

52. Tedesco FJ, Corless JK, Brownstein RE: Rectal sparing in antibiotic-associated pseudomembranous colitis. *Gastroenterology.* 1982;83:1259-1260.

53. DeGirolami PC, Hanff PA, Eichelberger K, et al. Multicenter evaluation of a new enzyme immunoassay for detection of *Clostridium difficile* enterotoxin A. *J Clin Microbiol.* 1992; 30:1085-1088.

54. Doern GV, Coughlin RT, Wu L. Laboratory diagnosis of *Clostridium difficile*-associated gastrointestinal disease: comparison of a monoclonal antibody enzyme immunoassay for toxins A and B with a monoclonal antibody enzyme immunoassay for toxin A only and two cytotoxicity assays. *J Clin Microbiol.* 1992;30:2042-2046.

55. Brazier JS. The diagnosis of *Clostidium difficile*-associated disease. *J Antimicrob Chemother.* 1998;41(suppl C):29-40.

56. Gerding DN, Johnson S, Peterson LR, et al. *Clostridium difficile*-associated diarrhea and colitis. *Infect Cont Hosp Epidemiol.* 1995;16:459-477.

57. Borriello SP, Vale T, Brazier JS, et al. Evaluation of a commercial enzyme immunoassay kit for the detection of *Clostridium difficile* toxin A. *Eur J Clin Microbiol Infect Dis.* 1992;11:360-363.

58. Wilcox MH. *Clostridium difficile* infection: appendix. *J Antimicrob Chemother.* 1998;41(suppl C):71-72.

59. Aronsson B, Mollby R, Nord CE. Diagnosis and epidemiology of *Clostridium difficile* enterocolitis in Sweden. *J Antimicrob Chemother.* 1984;14(suppl D):85-95.

60. Lyerly DM, Barroso LA, Wilkins TD. Identification of the latex test-reactive protein of *Clostridium difficile* as glutamate dehydrogenase. *J Clin Microbiol.* 1991;29:2639-2642.

61. George WL, Sutter VL, Citron D, et al. Selective and differential medium for isolation of *Clostridium difficile*. *J Clin Microbiol.* 1979;9:214-219.

62. Aspinall ST, Hutchinson DN. New selective medium for isolating *Clostridium difficile* from faeces. *J Clin Pathol.* 1992;45:812-814.

63. Bartley SL, Dowell VR Jr. Comparison of media for the isolation of *Clostridium difficile* from fecal specimens. *Lab Med.* 1991;22:335-338.

64. Kelly CP, Pothoulakis C, LaMont JT. *Clostridium difficile* colitis. *N Engl J Med.* 1994;330:257-262.

65. Gerding DN, Brazier JS. Optimal methods for identifying *Clostridium difficile* infections. *Clin Infect Dis.* 1993;16(suppl 4):S439-S442.

66. Nachamkin I, Lotz-Nolan L, Skalina D. Evaluation of a commercial cytotoxicity assay for detection of *Clostridium difficile* toxin. *J Clin Microbiol.* 1986;23:954-955.

67. Wren B, Clayton C, Tabaqchali S. Rapid identification of toxigenic *Clostridium difficile* strains by polymerase chain reaction. *Lancet.* 1990;335:423.

68. Kato N, Ou C-Y, Kato H, et al. Identification of toxigenic *Clostridium difficile* by the polymerase chain reaction. *J Clin Microbiol.* 1991;29:33-37.

69. McMillin DE, Muldrow LL, Laggette SJ, et al. Simultaneous detection of toxin A and toxin B genetic determinants of *Clostridium difficile* using the multiplex polymerase chain reaction. *Can J Microbiol.* 1992;38:81-83.

70. Shanholtzer CJ, Peterson LR, Olson MM, et al. Prospective study of gram-stained stool smears in diagnosis of *Clostridium difficile* colitis. *J Clin Microbiol.* 1983;17:906-908.

71. Levine HG, Kennedy M, LaMont JT. Counterimmunoelectrophoresis vs. cytotoxicity for the detection of *Clostridium difficile* toxin. *J Infect Dis*. 1982;145:398.

72. Madan E, Slifkin M. Stool caproic acid for screening of *Clostridium difficile*. *Am J Clin Pathol*. 1988;89:525-527.

73. Knoop FC, Owens M, Crocker IC. *Clostridium difficile*: clinical disease and diagnosis. *Clin Microbiol Rev*. 1993;6:257-265.

74. Triadafilopoulos G, Hallstone AE. Acute abdomen as the first presentation of pseudomembranous colitis. *Gastroenterology*. 1991;101:685-691.

75. Lipsett PA, Samantaray DK, Tam ML, et al. Pseudomembranous colitis: a surgical disease? *Surgery*. 1994;116:491-496.

76. Chatila W, Manthous CA. *Clostridium difficile* causing sepsis and an acute abdomen in critically ill patients. *Crit Care Med*. 1995;23:1146-1150.

77. Dignan CR, Greenson JK. Can ischemic colitis be differentiated from *C. difficile* colitis in biopsy specimens? *Am J Surg Pathol*. 1997;21:706-710.

78. Gerding DN. Diagnosis of *Clostridium difficile*-associated disease: patient selection and test perfection. *Am J Med*. 1996;100:485-486.

79. Cone JB, Wetzel W. Toxic megacolon secondary to pseudomembranous colitis. *Dis Colon Rectum*. 1982; 25:478-482.

80. Teasley DG, Gerding DN, Olson MM, et al. Prospective randomized trial of metronidazole versus vancomycin for *Clostridium difficile*-associated diarrhea and colitis. *Lancet*. 1983; 2:1043-1046.

81. Wenisch C, Parschalk B, Hasenhundl M, et al. Comparison of vancomycin, teicoplanin, metronidazole, and fusidic acid for the treatment of *Clostridium difficile*-associated diarrhea. *Clin Infect Dis*. 1996;22:813-818.

82. Young GP, Ward PB, Bayley N, et al. Antibiotic-associated colitis due to *Clostridium difficile*: double-blind comparison of vancomycin with bacitracin. *Gastroenterology*. 1985; 89:1038-1045.

83. Olson MM, Shanholtzer MT, Lee JT Jr, Gerding DN. Ten years of prospective *Clostridium difficile*-associated disease surveillance and treatment at the Minneapolis VA Medical Center. 1982-1991. *Infect Control Hosp Epidemiol*. 1994; 5:371-381.

84. Kleinfeld DI, Sharpe RJ, Donta ST. Parenteral therapy for antibiotic-associated pseudomembranous colitis. *J Infect Dis*. 1988;157:389.

85. Bolton RP, Culshaw MA. Fecal metronidazole concentrations during oral and intravenous therapy for antibiotic-associated colitis due to *Clostridium difficile*. *Gut*. 1986;27:1169-1172.

86. Dever LL, Smith SM, Handwerger S, Eng RH. Vancomycin-dependent *Enterococcus faecium* isolated from stool following oral vancomycin therapy. *J Clin Microbiol*. 1995;33:2770-2773.

87. Gerding DN, Johnson S, Peterson LR, et al. *Clostridium difficile*-associated diarrhea and colitis. *Infect Control Hosp Epidemiol*. 1995;16:459-477.

88. DeLalla F, Nicolin R, Rinaldi E, et al. Prospective study of oral teicoplanin versus oral vancomycin for therapy of pseudomembranous colitis and *Clostridium*-associated diarrhea. *Antimicrob Agents Chemother*. 1992;36:2192-2196.

89. Young G, McDonald M. Antibiotic-associated colitis: why do patients relapse? *Gastroenterology*. 1986;90:1098-1099.

90. Johnson S, Adelmann A, Clabots CR, et al. Recurrences of *Clostridium difficile* diarrhea not caused by the original infecting organism. *J Infect Dis*. 1989;159:340-343.

91. Fekety R, McFarland LV, Surawicz CM, et al. Recurrent *Clostridium difficile* diarrhea: charac-

teristics of and risk factors for patients enrolled in a prospective, randomized, double-blind trial. *Clin Infect Dis.* 1997;24:324-330.

92. O'Neill GL, Beaman MH, Riley TV. Relapse versus reinfection with *Clostridium difficile*. *Epidemiol Infect.* 1991;107:627-635.

93. Cleary RK. *Clostridium difficile*-associated diarrhea and colitis: clinical manifestations, diagnosis, and treatment. *Dis Colon Rectum.* 1998;41:1435-1449.

94. Tedesco FJ, Gordon D, Fortson WC. Approach to patients with multiple relapses of antibiotic-associated pseudomembranous colitis. *Am J Gastroenterol.* 1985;80:867-868.

95. Buggy BP, Fekety R, Silva J Jr. Therapy of relapsing *Clostridium difficile*-associated diarrhea and colitis with the combination of vancomycin and rifampin. *J Clin Gastroenterol.* 1987;9:155-159.

96. Moncino MD, Falleta JM. Multiple relapses of *Clostridium difficile*-associated diarrhea in a cancer patient: successful control with long term cholestyramine therapy. *Am J Pediatr Hematol Oncol.* 1992;14:361-364.

97. Kreutzer EW, Milligan FD. Treatment of antibiotic associated pseudomembranous colitis with cholestyramine resin. *John Hopkins Med J.* 1978;143:67-72.

98. Taylor MS, Bartlett JG. Binding of *Clostridium difficile* cytotoxin and vancomycin by anion exchange resins. *J Infect Dis.* 1980;141:92-97.

99. Surawicz CM, McFarland LV, Elmer G, Chin J. Treatment of recurrent *Clostridium difficile* colitis with vancomycin and *Saccharomyces boulardii*. *Am J Gastroenterol.* 1989; 84:1285-1287.

100. McFarland LV, Surawicz CM, Greenberg RN, et al. Prevention of beta-lactam-associated diarrhea by *Saccharomyces boulardii* compared with placebo. *Am J Gastroenterol.* 1995;90:439-448.

101. Castagluiolo I, Riegler MF, Valenick L, et al. *Saccharomyces boulardii* protease inhibits the effects of *Clostridium difficile* toxin A and B in human colonic mucosa. *Infect Immun.* 1999;67:302-307.

102. Gorbach SL, Chang T-W, Goldin B. Successful treatment of relapsing *Clostridium difficile* colitis with lactobacillus GG. *Lancet.* 1987;2:1519.

103. Biller JA, Katz AJ, Flores AF, et al. Treatment of recurrent *Clostridium difficile* colitis with lactobacillus GG. *J Pediatr Gastroenterol Nutr.* 1995;21:224-226.

104. Tvede M, Rask-Madsen J. Bacteriotherapy for chronic relapsing *Clostridium difficile* diarrhea in six patients. *Lancet.* 1989;1:1156-1160.

105. Schwan A, Sjolin S, Trottestam U, Aronsson B. Relapsing *Clostridium difficile* enterocolitis cured by rectal infusion of normal feces. *Scand J Infect Dis.* 1984;16:211-215.

106. Seal D, Borriello SP, Barclay F, et al. Treatment of relapsing *Clostridium difficile* diarrhea by administration of a non-toxigenic strain. *Eur J Clin Microbiol.* 1987;6:51-53.

107. Lewenstein A, Frigerio G, Moroni M. Biological properties of SF 68: a new approach for the treatment of diarrhoeal diseases. *Curr Ther Res.* 1979;26:967-981.

108. Siitonen S, Vapaataio H, Salminen S, et al. Effect of *Lactobacillus* GG yoghurt in prevention of antibiotic associated diarrhoea. *Ann Med.* 1990;22:57-59.

109. Schellenberg D, Bonington A, Champion CM, et al. Treatment of *Clostridium difficile* diarrhoea with brewer's yeast. *Lancet.* 1994;343:171-172.

110. Hassett J, Meyers S, McFarland L, Mulligan ME. Recurrent *Clostridium difficile* infection in a patient with selective IgG1 deficiency treated with intravenous immune globulin and *Saccharomyces boulardii*. *Clin Infect Dis.* 1995;20(suppl 2):266-268.

111. Kelly CP, Pothoulakis C, Vavva F, et al. Anti-*Clostridium difficile* bovine immunoglobulin concentrate inhibits cytotoxicity and enterotoxicity of *C. difficile* toxins. *Antimicrob Agents Chemother.* 1996;40:373-379.

112. Kelly CP, Chetham S, Keates S, et al. Survival of anti-*Clostridium difficile* bovine immunoglobulin concentrate in the human gastrointestinal tract. *Antimicrob Agents Chemother.* 1997;41:236-241.

113. Leung DYM, Kelly CP, Boguniewicz M, et al. Treatment with intravenously administered gamma globulin of chronic relapsing colitis induced by *Clostridium difficile* toxin. *J Pediatr.* 1991;118:633-637.

114. Medich DS, Lee KK, Simmons RL, et al. Laparotomy for fulminant pseudomembranous colitis. *Arch Surg.* 1992;127:847-852.

115. Morris JB, Zollinger RM Jr, Stellato TA. Role of surgery in antibiotic-induced pseudomembranous enterocolitis. *Am J Surg.* 1990;160:535-539.

116. McFarland LV, Mulligan M, Kwok RYY, Stamm WE. Nosocomial acquisition of *Clostridium difficile* infection. *N Engl J Med.* 1989;320:204-210.

117. Struelens MJ, Maas A, Nonhoff C, et al. Control of nosocomial transmission of *Clostridium difficile* based on sporadic case surveillance. *Am J Med.* 1991;91(suppl 3B):1385-1445.

118. Settle CD. *Clostridium difficile.* *Br J Hosp Med.* 1996;56:398-400.

119. Tabaqchali S, Jumaa P. Diagnosis and management of *Clostridium difficile* infection. *BMJ.* 1995;310:1375-1380.

120. Nolan NPM, Kelly CP, Humphreys JFH, et al. An epidemic of pseudomembranous colitis: importance of person-to-person spread. *Gut.* 1987;28:1467-1473.

121. Delmee M, Vandercam B, Avesani V, Michaux JL. Epidemiology and prevention of *Clostridium difficile* infections in a leukemia unit. *Eur J Clin Microbiol.* 1987;6:623-627.

122. Bender BS, Bennett R, Laughon BE, et al. Is *Clostridium difficile* endemic in chronic-care facilities? *Lancet.* 1986;2:11-13.

123. Ho M, Yang D, Wyle FA, Mulligan ME. Increased incidence of *Clostridium difficile*-associated diarrhea following decreased restriction of antibiotic use. *Clin Infect Dis.* 1996;23(suppl 1):102-106.

124. Kreisel D, Savel TG, Cunningham JD. Surgical antibiotic prophylaxis and *Clostridium difficile* toxin positivity. *Arch Surg.* 1995;130:989-993.

125. Brown E, Talbot GM, Axelrod P, et al. Risk factors for *Clostridium difficile* toxin-associated diarrhea. *Infect Control Hosp Epidemiol.* 1990;11:283-290.

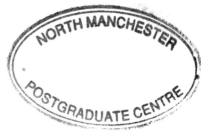

Donald E. Fry, MD, Professor and Chairman, University of New Mexico School of Medicine, Albuquerque, New Mexico, USA.